HYGGE

Discover Secrets to Managing a Fast Lifestyle and Introduce Unending Happiness to Your Home With Art of Hygge

(How to Enjoy Life Pleasures in the Simplicity of the Minimalist Lifestyle)

Robert Wagner

Published By Elena Holly

Robert Wagner

All Rights Reserved

Hygge: Discover Secrets to Managing a Fast Lifestyle and Introduce Unending Happiness to Your Home With Art of Hygge (How to Enjoy Life Pleasures in the Simplicity of the Minimalist Lifestyle)

ISBN 978-1-77485-357-3

Legal & Disclaimer

The information contained in this book is not designed to replace or take the place of any form of medicine or professional medical advice. The information in this book has been provided for educational and entertainment purposes only.

The information contained in this book has been compiled from sources deemed reliable, and it is accurate to the best of the Author's knowledge; however, the Author cannot guarantee its accuracy and validity and cannot be held liable for any errors or omissions. Changes are periodically made to this book. You must consult your doctor or get professional medical advice before using any of the suggested remedies, techniques, or information in this book.

Upon using the information contained in this book, you agree to hold harmless the Author from and against any damages, costs, and expenses, including any legal fees potentially resulting from the application of any of the information provided by this guide. This disclaimer applies to any damages or injury caused by the use and application, whether directly or indirectly, of any advice or information presented, whether for breach of contract, tort, negligence, personal injury, criminal intent, or under any other cause of action.

You agree to accept all risks of using the information presented inside this book. You need to consult a professional medical practitioner in order to ensure you are both able and healthy enough to participate in this program.

TABLE OF CONTENTS

Introduction

The next chapters will explore various advantages of incorporating the concept of Hygge throughout your day. If you're sick of being constantly in a hurry constantly and feeling that you're not welcome and there's an escape for you in our modern society Perhaps it's time to consider the concept of Hygge. If you adopt this approach you'll learn to slow down your pace and also learn to appreciate the small things in life, take time with the people you cherish, and focus on what is essential. This book will spend some time looking through Hygge and the implications it might mean for your life.

In this guidebook in this guidebook, we will discuss the basic concepts that are associated with the concept of Hygge. We will discuss the main elements of Hygge and the various concepts associated from this particular school of thought. Then, we will look at ways to incorporate the concept of Hygge into your daily routine. We will explore ways you can incorporate this to your daily life in your home and your relationships and even in the space where you work.

Hygge might be a concept that originates out of the Danish people however it is an idea that is utilized across the globe. If you're looking to live a life complete with comfort, relaxation and warm feelings which make you be more relaxed, make sure you read this book and discover all there is to know about Hygge.

There are many books on the subject available that are available, thank you to you for picking this one! We have made every effort to ensure that it's packed with as much valuable information as could be. We hope you enjoy!

Chapter 1: What's Hygge, and Where Did It Come from?

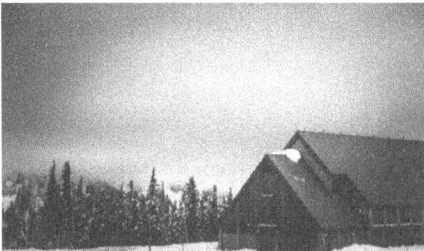

Hygge is commonly called an Danish word. But it was actually born as a word in Old Norwegian tongue. The closest translation for the word in its original form today is 'well-being'.

It was adopted into Danish culture at the late 18th century, and is now part of their language.

Nowadays, the word is frequently used. However, it's much more than just a phrase. Hygge is a term that a lot of Danes utilize on a daily basis. People use the term "Hygge for many things. It can be confusing if you travel to Denmark and aren't aware of the meaning behind it.

It is important to remember that this idea has been in use for a number of years. Since 2016, it has gained an online popularity as a lifestyle choice However, this isn't true.

It's not a secret that the Danish are thought to be among the most joyful people on earth and this is evident in the term Hygge.

"Hygge" is the word used to describe a feeling. Hygge is pronounced Hue-Guh . it's used to refer to specific occasions that occur in the course of your day. The best moments are those when you are satisfied and content. The perfect moment could be spent with your others. You could be cuddling up at your home or in the middle of a wild celebration. However, whenever you have something that feels warm and unique, the experience is Hygge.

There isn't a literal translation to English The meaning is loosely translated as comfort and happiness which emphasizes that it is more of a feeling than physical. This means that it is different for each person.

Hygge is a cult concept in Denmark because it's a great way to see the good even in the most difficult of times. For instance, Denmark is known to have long and harsh winters. even in winter there's just seven hours of sunlight per day, which is about seventeen hours in darkness.

Finding Hygge is a way to reduce mental health issues since there is a sense of gratitude for the little aspects of life.

This is vital; Hygge is not a style of living that must be embraced You can't purchase Hygge-themed food items or furniture. It's just a way of feeling that you enjoy and constantly seek out. It's why it's possible to integrate it into your daily routine and increase your perspective about the world. It's also possible to experience a hygge moment at any time.

The practice of incorporating hygge into the daily routine involves figuring out how to make everyday routines feel unique. One of the easiest examples is making your morning cup of coffee or tea. It's not about turning on the kettle or the coffee maker. You want to establish a routine that turns it into an unforgettable moment in your day.

It could mean moving away from the traditional method of making tea, and instead adopting an Chinese method, or making the tea in a pot, and using genuine porcelain cups as well as saucers. Also, it could be a matter of using a filter coffee machine , as well as the "good" cups.

The hygge way of living doesn't mean you have to invest a large sum in redecorating or getting rid of everything you own. All you have to learn is to spot and appreciate Hygge moments within your routine.

When you're aware of the kind of occasions are, or the capacity to be Hygge, you'll realize that it's a part of many of your routines.

Of sure, there are plenty of books on hygge or lifestyle guides, and even restaurants that are themed around Scandinavia. But, you don't have to need all of them.

This book will help you understand how to find Hygge in your life and ways you can implement it into your life. This will allow you to find more harmony in your life, and be more satisfied. That's a huge accomplishment in today's economy and social situation.

This is perhaps the most appealing feature of hygge: it doesn't matter which rut you're stuck in and how hard life can be or even in the event that you're experiencing financial hardship. Finding, and embracing the concept of hygge throughout your day can transform your outlook, and even your life.

It's crucial to remember that hygge does not mean buying a teapot; cozy throws, or a variety of candles. It's not about creating some hygge experiences in your daily life. They already are there. What you have to find them is to accept them.

It is said that hygge can be described as a mindset that people with terminal illness usually adopt, even when they're not aware of it. Patients diagnosed with terminal illness begin to take in every day life and see the everyday as exceptional.

This is what you'll be taught, you'll learn that all things you do can be praised as exceptional even though it's not. Hygge will help you appreciate for everything in your life that are truly important.

When you first start it's important to consider hygge and seek out those moments. In time, this becomes a normal routine. You won't be looking for hygge. You'll observe it in all of your activities.

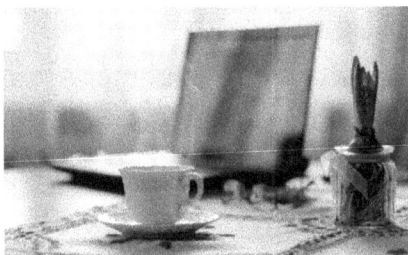

At this point, it's a continuation of your regular routine and will help you see the world as enjoyable, not a stressful experience or something you just must get through.

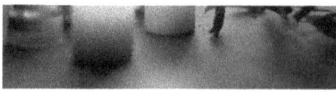

It is important to note that although Hygge is all about being present but it's much more than this. It's not just about having to stay present; but also should let yourself be in the present moment, even though it appears to be a minor or perhaps insignificant ceremony to people who don't know.

It doesn't matter what phase of your life or what challenges you're dealing with. There is hygge even in the smallest of details and even in the most impressive achievements. All you need to do is determine what you're seeking. After that, you'll be able to live your life in a more fulfilling and satisfying way.

Chapter 2: Benefits of Hygge

Hygge might not be an actual way of life in the same manner as being an Buddhist or a nomadic. But the incorporation of it into your lifestyle can provide a variety of advantages.

Improved Mental Health

Hygge perfectly embodies the Danes attitude towards long, cold winters. They are positive and find reasons to be happy. This will help keep them from feeling depressed in these dark, long winter months.

There's no need to endure seventeen hours of dark each day to appreciate how hygge is able to help you feel more

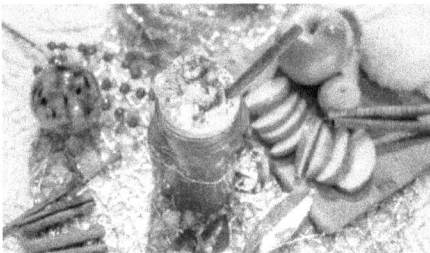

optimistic about your life.

If you're someone who tends to think about things for a long time and things that are not yours, a search for hygge within your everyday life will allow you let go. This will reduce the amount of time you spend at home, which reduces the chance of sinking into depression.

Being active in your mind can help prevent cognitive problems as you age. But a mind that is constantly focused on negative issues can lead to stress levels and cause feeling of overwhelm.

Just embracing one thing in each day to make it extraordinary will aid in breaking this pattern and avoid feeling overwhelmed. This can make a massive positive impact on your mental wellbeing.

Naturally, just taking in the moment can mean that you'll let go of all of the things that are now causing you stress. This gives your mind the chance to relax and prevent mental health issues that are gaining momentum.

Self-worth and confidence increase

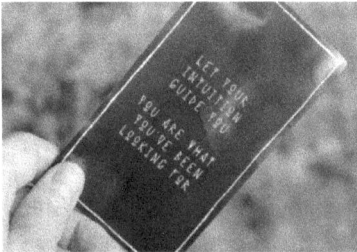

Self-worth is the way you judge your worth. The more you are proud of your actions, the higher your self-worth. It is important to note that higher self-esteem levels are associated with the belief that you deserve to be treated with respect.

It shouldn't be an unsurprising fact that those who believe they deserve to be respected are generally received with respect. That's because if not respected, they will never interact with someone else.

It's an excellent way to earn respect. It will also boost your confidence. If people are influenced by your higher self-esteem, they'll be more likely to take your thoughts into consideration and implement your suggestions into procedures in the future.

There's no magic trick involved. If you display confidence and self-esteem, people will think you're knowledgeable about and will listen. When they see that you are aware of what you're talking about , they'll pay more attention.

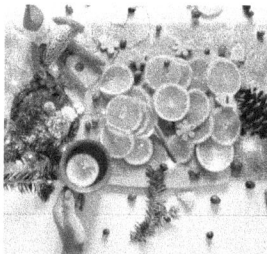

Enhancing your confidence and success in life begins with acknowledging your self-worth.

Hygge can help with this. One of the most effective methods to boost self-esteem is to accomplish things. When you succeed, you are happy about yourself and the ability to accomplish more. This improves your feelings of self-worth when you realize that you can contribute to contribute in every situation.

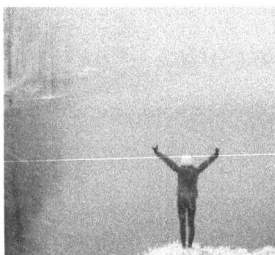

The good thing is that success starts with a simple. Set yourself the goal of reading for 30 minutes per day in reading. It's fairly simple and is achievable. Once you've completed it for a week , you can celebrate the accomplishment as an exceptional occasion. Your self-esteem will increase and in turn your confidence.

It's also important to note that when you're comfortable in a particular situation or within your own body , you're more likely to to connect with other people. This will increase your social circle and increase the opportunities that are available to you. There's a chance that a new friend might have a new exciting possibility for you, regardless of whether you've dreamed of it, or perhaps not.

Lower stress/better health

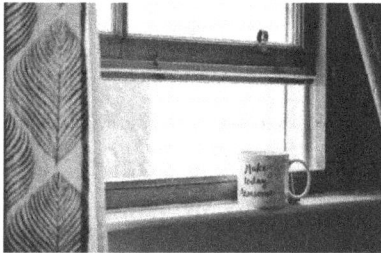

Stress is risky, yet it's an essential part of our lives. If you're stressed, the body produces a chemical known as cortisol. This hormone blocks the production of many other hormones your body produces.

Cortisol's job is to help you prepare to either fight or flee. It's an instinctive response which is sometimes essential. In most cases, running away or fighting aren't realistic alternatives. For instance, when your boss asks you to join for a daily meeting.

However, since the body can't identify the various forms of stress. Therefore, it releases cortisol each time.

However, research has shown that chronic stress can contribute to the formation of numerous age-related diseases. This includes Alzheimer's, cancer and cardiovascular problems.

Stress reduction is crucial to maintain your health and longevity. Any activity that helps you to be in the moment will help reduce stress. Hygge encourages you to embrace a moment as extraordinary. As a result you'll be able to forget the other issues happening in your daily life.

Take this along with the pleasure of relaxing in a moment of hygge and stress levels will drop.

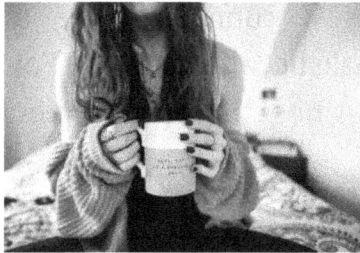

There are many ways to lessen stress, including checking your diet, exercising regularly, and staying clear of stressful situations. However, the practice of embracing hygge can do more than simply reduce stress levels. It allows you to be more relaxed and enjoy every time in your life. It releases endorphins that help you feel more relaxed and lessen discomfort, both physical and psychological.

In the end, achieving the right time to relax will allow reduce anxiety and increase your potential for health.

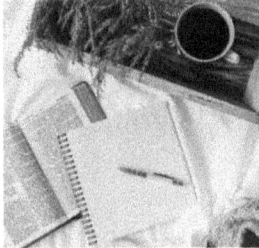

There's no guarantee in this world, but if even something as simple as Hygge can benefit you, it's something worthwhile to embrace. It's also important to note that reducing stress can reduce the risk of comfort eating or eating out, assisting you keep the weight you are at. It also helps reduce dependence on other methods of coping including alcohol or drugs.

It will also boost your health and outlook but it can also be beneficial to your pocketbook.

Better balance between life and work

Another major advantage of hygge practice is that it helps you to maintain a balance between your work and personal life. Once you begin looking for moments of hygge within your daily life, you'll begin to realize what's significant, and what's not.

This will alter your thinking and your perspective on your daily life. While work is an essential aspect of our lives, it should not be the only thing you do. Making a routine that brings you home on time each day will allow you to be less stressed as well as spend time more with the people you cherish.

This is crucial as research has shown that when your balance between work and life isn't right, everybody around you is affected. You're more likely to become unhappy, feel stressed and take irrational choices. This could have a devastating impact on the people in your vicinity.

Because hygge is a way to bring joy even in the smallest details and you'll be able to spend more time on the things that are simple. More importantly having more fun with small details can help you to relax and have fun more.

It will actually enhance your relationship with the people close to you. This has the positive effect, making it more enjoyable for you to be around them which will improve your time-to-work/life balance.

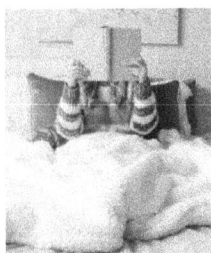

Being present in the moment doesn't mean trying to find something more satisfying. In other words, you will begin to appreciate the things you already have.

That's the kind of perspective that usually occurs with age however, it can be achieved through the introduction of hygge into your daily life.

More mindfulness

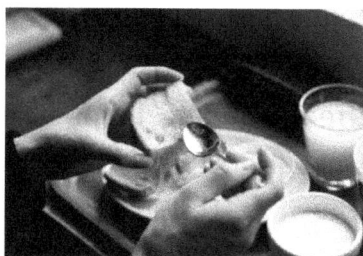

If you're rushing from one thing to the next, and you do not feel that you have time to slow down and relax Hygge will be able help you.

Mindfulness can be described as internal concentration, which allows you to be more conscious of your feelings as well as thoughts in a certain moment in time. However, it's not just simply being aware of your own thoughts and should increase your awareness to the involvement of other people within your life.

When you are aware, you'll be able to appreciate the joy that little things can give. Also, you'll appreciate the loved people who are in your life more.

The best part is that there is no need to devote all day meditating. The ability to be more conscious of what's happening around you can be accomplished by contemplating the idea of hygge, and then recognizing the concept in your day life. By embracing hygge, you can take pleasure in a beverage of tea or coffee, relish the aroma of a cake and, perhaps most important enjoy every moment that you spend with another person.

When you realize the benefits of taking time to enjoy the moment, you'll see your outlook on life changing. It is possible to continue working and succeed while enjoying the hygge.

Instead of constantly busy it is important to take time to do the simple things, and really appreciate these things. It will take time but the reward isn't only taking care of your surroundings and your own needs.

The Danes have proven that taking regular breaks help to give you new perspectives, increasing your productivity and creative.

For instance what number of times have you noticed that having an unplanned break from a difficult issue makes you find the solution? Hygge-based practices encourage this!

It is also important to note that the increase in mindfulness can help you to recognize the real value of the things that just seem important. This new perspective can help to ensure that you have a clear plan of action and will feel more in charge of your life.

Don't forgetthat hygge relaxes the mind, eliminates the haze of anger or frustration and makes you more peacefully and, consequently, healthier.

Beware of being deceived to believe that making time for coffee can bring hygge into your life, and alter everything. It's not about what you're doing, but how you're doing it that's important.

It is easy to use

One of the benefits of hygge is it is easy to incorporate into your daily routine. There aren't any complicated dietary demands to follow. There is no need to reorganize your furniture or buy new furniture or accessories that conform to a certain design Hygge isn't just about the surroundings, but rather about making time to you and sharing your time with other people.

The location you choose to use during this time is irrelevant. To create the perfect atmosphere, it's important to have a comfortable space. However, you'll be amazed by how cozy a room feels when you turn off the lights and curl up with someone you cherish.

Hygge is simple to incorporate into your everyday life. Once you have a grasp of the idea of hygge, you can follow this guide to incorporate it into your daily routine.

While your attitude is what matters, you are able to alter your home's layout in order to make it easier for you to enjoy and capture these moments.

We'll offer suggestions for how to accomplish this in the following chapter. Be aware that this is a personal issue and what works for one person may not be the case for you. Consider what triggers your mindful moment when you are considering changing the furniture at home.

More Optimistic

It could be surprising, but recognizing and identifying Hygge moments in your day could actually boost your confidence.

Like we said, taking an hour of hygge lets you unwind from the constant snoring happening. In most cases, this can lead to a solution to an issue. The reason you're able to identify the solution is because you've taken a take a step back and look at the bigger perspective.

The more time you spend doing this, the more possibilities you'll discover for solving the current issues. This will create confidence in you believing that you will come up with a solution if you tackle an issue in the right way.

This optimism will show up in your daily routine. You'll notice that you're more positive in every situation.

This is perhaps the fact about Hygge. It's easy to incorporate into your daily routine, but it could have an impact on the activities you are currently doing and would like to accomplish. The reason for this is that Hygge lets you see what you truly would like to achieve. Once you've established what's important to you, it's easier to set and attain objectives.

This is the secret to happiness and it's a lot easier to attain than you think.

Chapter 3: Hygge Home & Furniture

The beginning of your life will be the one that is the most precious to the personal space of your home that is your home. We are planning to transform your home into a sanctuary of tranquility and pleasure. It's just made so much sense to begin our journey here, because your home is our personal space. Everyone would want to make it as peaceful and serene as they can, wouldn't we?

Then, where do you start?

It's actually the toughest aspect, as it is likely that you'll be overwhelmed and it's not going to be on the notion of Hygge. The issue is that many most people view their whole house (and everything else in their home) in one go however this is not the case.

We'll help you figure out the most effective way to deal with the house, since it's much easier than you might think at this moment. With this in mind, here is what we're going to accomplish.

Start by taking just one space. In this instance we'll be taking your living area. But, the same rules and procedures are applicable to any room within your home.

First, be patient and take in the space. Examine every corner, each item and the location of the items, the lights and the power they have. Sit in the center of the room and take note of each area. After that, move around and observe things from various angles, so that you can gain an idea of what things look like from various angles.

The most important thing to keep in mind is that hygge is a personal experience to you. It's the state of mind that you are in and obviously, it is a matter of personal preference. inside our home. Rooms have different sizes and different fixtures can't be removed. Also, this is just a reference and not instructions for each task you must accomplish in your home.

Why do you have to take this step? Why should you be observing every room this way before beginning? It may seem absurd initially.

It's actually quite simple to comprehend. To better grasp of the current situation this, we'll take you through a variety of ways you can take at the moment to bring a touch of the hygge into every space. We will discuss each one of them.

1. Declutter

The accumulation of stuff that has no purpose (aside of collecting dust) is a big no-no for the notion of the concept of hygge. This is such a crucial element that we actually have an entire section on decluttering, and how to go about doing it. We will get into more detail later however we need to say removal of items which have no purpose to exist is an integral element of bringing the concept of hygge in your home.

2. Consider the comfort

We've said repeatedly that comfort is synonymous with Hygge and therefore it is logical to think about ways to create a more relaxing space. We know that comfort isn't a simple word to define since, again it is a personal thing to each person.

With this in mind, here are the most important things to consider on this topic.

* Comfort is related to the ability to be relaxed in a room

If you notice that something doesn't seem or feel comfortable to you, you should make it right.

* Make sure the room isn't too hot or cold, as this is not exactly a sign of comfort.

The warmth, feeling cozy and snug is the target, even if you are located in the corner

3. Think about creating the Hyggekrog

So, you're considering the term Hyggekrog. It is likely that you will be a bit confused about what exactly it means but the solution is very simple. The basic meaning of this concept is to: "being in a location that you can find a place in your house that is likely to be near a window or somewhere relaxing and tranquil to look at and get enthralled by the concept of the word hygge'. In normal English the word hygge means a warm space.

Most people will look at adding cushions, maybe a blanket with fur, and then just relax in the moment while enjoying a warm drink. If you also are able to have a fire going or candles behind you, you're taking hygge inside your home to an entirely new level.

4. Remember the candles

Since we've talked about candles, let's discuss them for a second. The soothing effect of candles can't be overestimated regardless of whether they're scented or not. The presence of candles in your space is a must for those who enjoy hygge.

I prefer to spread them across the space to provide the illusion of a soft source of light as well as a relaxing effect from burning flames. This is a typical usage is to do this in Scandinavia where there are often shorter days and longer nights particularly during winter.

5. Be aware of the natural world around you.

Nature is another major element of hygge because we Scandinavian individuals are so in touch to our environment. We are not very fond of urban environments in this area. We enjoy spending time to the forest! It is highly recommended to find ways to incorporate your nature into the space.

This can be accomplished in many ways however one of the most important is to make sure you have as many wooden furniture pieces as feasible. In the end using any natural substance for furniture is a good idea. Anything else to wooden (of every kind) can be considered to be anti-hygge, and is something you should stay clear of.

It is also worth using natural materials as well as plants in your rooms. Any thing that has the potential of bringing the outdoors into your home, and allow you to connect to nature somehow. It's more beneficial when the natural environment you invite into your home is vibrant and flourishing, naturally.

6. The proper placement of lamps

Although we've previously discussed the importance of candles, you might consider investing in lamps. With these lamps, we're talking about low-wattage and warm lightinstead of any bright light source, sInce the whole goal is to create some kind of glow around the area. It is perfectly acceptable to use energy-efficient LED lamps, as they've evolved to be very comfortable and hygge-friendly (read that a warm glow is also possible with environmentally friendly lamps!).

Consider their location. Put the lamps in an unlit space for a more lively look to the space. Place a lamp on a table near where you're sitting to gain some extra comfort by its light. If you are able, opt for lamps with different settingsso that you can adjust the intensity of the lighting. When the outside gets darker it is possible to dim the brightness inside to create that cozy feel.

7. Furniture should be useful

We're not talking just about the house generally and also the furniture. In the present, we're all guilty of accumulating furniture pieces and then adding more till our houses are bursting at the point. However, that's not the best situation to be in.

Furniture must function at all times. It should be able for use and it should not have any difficulties in doing this. The table that's stuck in the corner, and is only utilized when the rest of the room is moved isn't practical in the sense of Hygge. The process of getting it to a point that we are able to use it is both stressful and frustrating which are two feelings one must strive to stay clear of.

Don't be afraid to take out some furniture pieces to make space. Try arranging your space to make the most of the furniture pieces you already own. If you have to, consider reducing the size so you can make use of your furniture instead of it becoming a statue.

8. Remember those final touches

In the majority of cases, it is the finishing details that add a major impact to the interior of your home. Again, we can imagine a lounge and the best way to add these little details, and there are a myriad of options to choose from.

For instance, battery powered lighting is utilized in display units to provide an element of warmth. Utilizing the full potential of the fireplace, it makes it inviting and warm. Use of throws on the sofas to help break up the harshness and provide you with a cuddly thing to do. The rug with fur on the floor made of wood (since wood is the natural material) will give you an extra warm surface to rest your feet on. You must bring in things that bring you joy and that's the main important thing.

Chapter 4: Hygge Is Founded On the Principle of Simplicity

"Hygge" originates originated from the Old Norse word, "hugga" that is translated as "hoo-gah" meaning to console or provide comfort. It is also believed to be the origin for"hugg" in the English term "hug" meaning holding someone with an embrace that is warm. When you consider these two meanings, they suggest Hygge as a synonym for warmth, comfort and intimacy.

The Danish people are a bit different. Denmark, Hygge is more than just a term; it's an entire lifestyle. Many have attempted to comprehend what it means living in Hygge. It is one of the most talked about words of the present. People all over all over the world are seeking happiness, yet they aren't finding it. They Danish consider that the happiness can be located in the things exists already. It is the Hygge practice is the way they find the source of happiness.

The concept behind Hygge is to maximize the moments that are special and small everyday pleasures. It doesn't necessarily mean that someone gifted you with the latest car or an unexpected cut in your career, but these are events that are worth celebrating as well. An unforgettable moment could be as easy as a cold night with your loved ones at home and you are able to take a relaxing movie with hot chocolate, or simply laying with a blanket, talking.

In essence, the essence of a Hygge feeling is the total absence of things that would cause emotional stress or discomfort. When you are in this state you can relax and enjoy the simple and soothing things . You pamper yourself with items that give you joy and warmth.

In the world in which we are anxious and overwhelm, happiness is said to be expensive, and lots of it. If you're looking for a great escape, a relaxing spa or a relaxing day is going to cost you.

The Danes who practice Hygge don't need to pay anything to be calm, relaxed or happy. It is true that Hygge isn't a product that needs to be purchased and, in fact, it will not cost anything. It is an art form that is based on simplicity in the sense that the essentials you need to make it are not a burden to purchase.

In Hygge candles that are basic are preferred over expensive ones, a knitted blanket is preferred to a designer one, a homemade baked bread that's slightly burnt to a flavorful bread from the bakery, and hot beverages in a mug rather than a sweet latte.

If one is at ease with such things that aren't regarded high in society and they are content even with the most prestigious of them. That's without tying their happiness to the things they own, and even if they were to lose everything and reverted to simpler times just the things would be gone, not their joy.

If we're not tied to our possessions; which is the stuff that we own that we are attached to, we will have an opportunity to look around and appreciate the other benefits we enjoy that aren't tagged with price tags like friends, family health, peace, health whatever it is. You're right that a love affair and attachment to material objects can hinder us from recognizing these blessings.

Imagine someone who is in the pursuit of fashion and buying the latest fashions in bags or clothing. They might appear happy in the beginning, at least on Instagram or other social media where they have a platform to showcase their latest purchases. However, if you were to remove them from the expensive clothing or other items the person will be to be a shell. They are entangled with the item and might suffer from depression in the event that they fail to be able to afford the item. It is their life as well as other gifts. true gifts that don't take away from them, like family appear to be non-essential.

Hygge is a way to let go of sight and let go of these as blinding attachments. This is the reason it is based on simplicity being the lowest of the social ranks. You can afford a luxurious restaurant but instead you wear old sweatpants and have a sloppy breakfast by yourself with beloved family members. You can pay for the spa experience to be pampered but you decide to stay at back at home, soak in a relaxing bath in a nice warm temperature, flick on some candles, and enjoy a drink while you gaze at them shine - to take pleasure in the simplest things.

According to an Hygge enthusiast and the founder of Philadelphia located Hygge wellness fitness expert Samantha J. Vander Wielen describes Hygge as "Hygge is a perfect description of what is meant by being satisfied. It's not things that make us feel happy It's making the effort to find out what fills our tanks internally."

Hygge is not demanded or imposed

You cannot be able to force Hygge regardless of the amount of pastries, or pillows and throw blankets there are. You can certainly attempt to influence it, but you can't forcibly force it. It can also be triggered, prioritized or even facilitated.

Hygge is not without its own rules. It can happen, at times when it is facilitated, and sometimes it happens at the time you would least expect it. For example, if you experience a power outage on a winter night and you are in darkness and you need to ignite candles, set fire to and put on a blanket to stay warm because the electric heater has gone turned off. There's no television to distract you, and you might find yourself having the most wonderful conversation you've had for many years. This will be one of your most memorable shared memories.

Sometimes, a well-planned Hygge night could end up unsatisfactory. This is particularly true when we've set expectations too high, or have planned our event with such care. Perhaps Hygge doesn't like being pushed around or questioned.

Hygge is the time where you relax. You free yourself from constraints, expectations, stress and all distractions, and allow things to flow while you take pleasure in simple and relaxing moments like playing cards with your loved one, sharing stories of your childhood, or reading books together, and the list goes on.

Chapter 5: What is Hygge?

In the context of "hygge" (pronounced "hugge") there is unfortunately, no similar phrase in German language. It is possible to claim that the Danish"hygge" is a relaxing environment or feeling of relaxation. The word "hyggelig" literally refers to "pleasant", "cozy" and "nice" and was originally "carefully" as well as "thoughtful". However, over time it gained its meaning as "spreading health and well-being".

As we can discern, Hygge can have different implications, and they are positive. As per Meik Wiking, another author of the book, "An approach to life that brings you joy", Hygge is the art of creating a comfortable environment and discover joy in the smallest of things. We could ask an Dane what Hygge is, or what the word "Philosophy" means. What is the reason it has such a huge appeal, he'd smile, since Hygge is a normal lifestyle for everyone Danes. This is the reason why many are surprised that it is now a type of global export success all over the world. because being happy is all it takes to be happy to be happy, enjoy life and do things you are happy about. The author, who also published a book titled The greatest happiness is found in the smallest things Marie Tourell Soderberg, emphasizes that hygge is available everywhere. It's just a matter of knowing what to look out for.

Maybe a cup of tea or hot chocolate freshly prepared Listen to the sounds of rain from the window, snuggle up in your bed on a winter day, enjoy a meal with family and friends, and read those pages from a brand new book; hear the sounds of the fireplace or a blanket, freshly baked cake from the oven.

This and much more makes up Hygge, the Danish method of living. Maybe you've been practicing these kinds of practices for quite a while, but you didn't know about it having been given a name.

It's a concept which does not have an easy translation, even though many have been written recently. It's hard to find a term in Spanish that is simple in what it refers to because it is able to concentrate on the cozy from the sense of comfort, well-being, and even the freedom. It can be said as an expression that is seeking happiness at home by enjoying the simple things.

STEPS to GEL

There is no one who is as famous for their ability to live in harmony and be happy as Scandinavians and Danes specifically. So, it is only in Scandinavia that the phenomenon of hygge can be seen or, in Russian style, "huge". It is often not conveyed as comfort or coziness. To fully understand what it means it is, the authors suggest presenting Sunday evenings in a group of friends or family that you can feel calm as well as joy and happiness in your life. The authors say that according to them the Danes love that the hug is everywhere, at work and home. If not the average Dane won't be afflicted with the same stress on Sundays: meals with family and friends and on Monday mornings - the office is dull and boring. The authors are certain that a welcoming, warm and homey atmosphere will make working more enjoyable. But, is not the case. Dane is great. Do I really need the hygge look in an office in a Russian office? Perhaps it can be effective on work that is creative however not for the standard ones. In order to understand the concept of hygge authors provide practical and proven steps.

Techniques to understand the HYGGE

Favorite Mug

Choose a cup of coffee which you cherish. There's nothing better then sipping your cup of morning cup of coffee and discussing the latest news with a coworker. Also, during the morning, a few tea breaks can help your brain relax from the hum of the workplace.

Music Selection

A variety of enjoyable and relaxing instrumental music can be the perfect companion to your work day and can help alleviate tension. Remember that music is a great way to relax.

Oxygen Cocktail

Lunch break and a time to stop activities to allow relaxation to your body. avoid checking the social networks or mail and go outside in the fresh air to clear your mind. Eat and drink on the park bench, feeding the pigeons or simply watching other people. You will not be able to notice when you can get in a wonderful mood.

Home Workplace Environment

Why should work be comprised of boring furniture for cabinets as well as terminals and chairs that are uncomfortable? Bring slippers to home, place them on in a rocking chair and display photos of your loved relatives. Every day, bring flowers. Absolutely anything that breaks the rules of workplace routine (within the bounds of reason, of course). The Danes are a good example. They get enthralled by candles and put them in any place they can. Are you worse?

Joint Lunch with colleagues

Your lunch break can be transformed into a casual meal with your colleagues (again in a reasonable manner). Plan "feast" days and reward your colleagues to specially prepared meals to mark the celebration. In the end, it's not mean that food is an integral aspect of a hug. She can help you enjoy the moment and build friendship.

Doing good deeds with no reason

Remember the cartoon in which the characters would give flowers in answer to the question "for why?" They always said "But exactly like that." That's what they call the "hugge." Give the candy a treat or give someone you admire them and they will end the day happy even if, at the end that daytime, hasn't thought about it since the beginning of the day. The thought of having someone who will take care of you eases any anxiety.

The Team The Team All

The Danes are familiar with living in groups which is why they're always confident, regardless of their personal shortcomings and remain modest even when they are part of the authority. Hygge is a great method to boost the spirit of the group and create the feeling of ownership. Set up friendly competitions in the office or for individual events while on the go. For instance, invite your colleagues to join in bowling. Also, keep in mind that "hygge" doesn't mean a need to be perfect rather, it's a recognition of the importance of each day which is enjoyed. In the end, everything that is great in the world is comprised of a few crumbs.

What do the bosses expect from the bosses? Can they put the hygge concept to offer intangible rewards during a crisis? Add - again dependent upon the character of work and the personality of the manager.

Chapter 6: Hygge, The Danish Art Of Happiness

Hygge is known as "ugueu," comes directly from Denmark. It is definitely not something new since it is among the pillars of the Scandinavian lifestyle. This is probably the reason why Denmark is still the top nation that is the most happy on earth. It took just a bit of time to finally cross the border.

Even though there's not much sunlight in winter (the night is in the day) and the temperatures are more than freezing but the Danes were able to discover the way to achieve the ultimate happiness.

It's the how we arrange our homes or our routines for the day or the moments we have spent surrounded by loved ones, or even the words we use to express ourselves each aspect of our lives is important. Every aspect is designed to be enjoyable in the present moment. The

Danes have naturally implemented the Hygge practice of living from the time of their childhood.

They're looking for an individual experience that they want to be able to share with their family and friends. Hygge is a method of being, acting thoughts, eating, and living simply.

The Danes are a good example. They are aiming to transform their homes into comfortable, warm and practical place to be able to relax with their family. Objective: Simplicity.

Hygge therefore is a term that has many meanings based the way you interpret it. Many will be embracing this concept all the time, whether it's family events and special events, gatherings or celebrations, and even small meals. The objective is to find our comfortable zone.

Here's my interpretation of hygge:

1. Attention: There's nothing better than snuggling your body inside the blankets as you enjoy the rain, or watch those steamy bubbles. The idea of watching a show on TV with your friends is even more enjoyable. This is referred to as "hyggeling home."

2. Find time for yourself with new walks or meditations breaks for reading and playlists for relaxation or even writing as in my case. It's important to make time for yourself.

3. Recipe for homemade: Hygge is also a idea that can be enjoyed around the table. Have a nutritious dinner for two with your family, friends or your colleagues. Have fun cooking fresh ingredients.

4. A cozy space The idea is not to completely redo the entire house, but rather to modify the look. Utilize a table lamp create a warm light in your space, place the freshest flowers, or even plants inside the home and then use candles that

smell. It's worth it for peace and tranquility.

Six ways to embrace Hygge

Hygge (pronounced Hoo-Ga) is a lovely Danish idea that encourages people to take a moment of silence and let us be more present in our lives, and take time to nourish and appreciate the small and everyday things.

These are my best six ways to help you achieve this level:

1. Clean and restored

At Wild Nutrition We believe in the seasonal cleansing process, and the time to cleanse during the winter months is not any different (in fact, it's two days of the Wild Nutrition Total Cleansing program as I type this). A chance to replenish and nourish your body and mind prior to winter's arrival.

2. Reduce the time

The seasonally appropriate exercise that allows for the slow pace of winter. Imagine Yoga, light walking and walking on those cold winter mornings. Deep breathing and meditation can help you relax and aid in bringing the body to a state of parasympathetic. This is extremely helpful to reduce stress hormones and helping to improve digestion.

3. Put your money into candles

The glow of a candle is able to warm any space and create a mood. Candles can be part of a night-time ritual to signify the wind's arrival at the close to the workday. Make sure you choose candles that are not toxic to avoid polluting the indoor air. Our favorite candles are Neom and Beefayre.

4. Take it slow

Enjoy cooking slow while enjoying the smells and sharing your meals with family and family and friends. The digestive juices are actually increased when you smell of food, so you should take time when cooking and then consume the food to improve digestion.

5. Use a lot of spices and herbs that are warming.

Incorporate spices and herbs into your stews and soups to will improve digestion and circulation. Ginger and rosemary, black pepper horseradish, garlic, paprika cayenne pepper and cumin are deliciously nutritious.

6. Book that turns into a worm

Take advantage of the benefits of a good read for a healthy snack before heading to work or home and to relax in the evenings with reading e-mails and social networks. You'll be amazed how relaxed you are.

Here's How You Hygge (Your Way)

Perhaps you've been aware of the term hygge (pronounced HOO-gah) which is the

Danish style of living that emphasizes intimacy as well as all the other things that feel good. It's not just one thing, but rather a way to live your life in a more mindful relaxed, cozy, and hazy way. Think of cuddling in a cozy spot to read a novel, sipping warm mulled wine in front of the fireplace or having a delicious and filling meal with people you love.

A fundamental tenet in Danish culture for many centuries, Hygge has recently stormed the the world. It is partly due to the growing popularity of Scandinavian design and, possibly due to the joy of living in the midst that is filled with ever-growing Instagram routes and an endless news cycle.

It's a refreshing view of life in general and an opportunity to revel in the good things that are right, regardless of how small or big.

Be a part of the Light

To create the tranquility of hygge in your home, pay attention to providing adequate lighting. Make the most of natural light If you can, try raising your curtainsand setting a table close to a window and basking in the splendor of its shining. Because Denmark has extremely lengthy and dark winters that are dark and cold, artificial lighting is also important to incorporate, both through chandeliers and candles without scent. (Curiously It is estimated that Danes utilize on average 13 pounds of wax for each household during the course of a year.)

Discover beauty in the contrasts

The materials utilized in the creation of hygge can be a test of various variations. On one hand, there are your creations that are soft and comfortable such as big clothes, soft fabrics, quilts, flannel, as well as linen. In contrast, you have luxurious and smooth materials like ceramics, soft woods and marble. It's the contrast of soft and hard, crisp and warm that creates the equilibrium that Hygge is aiming to attain.

Cocoon in the intimate

Hygge helps with nesting, which means digging into an inviting and luxurious space in complete privacy. Get a pair woolen socks, a softer blanket and hyggebusker the sweatpants you love which won't be discovered dead outside your home.

Gather around

The social aspect plays a significant part in Hygge since there is a belief that pleasures of living a happy and healthy life can be best enjoyed with your people you know.

Try the flavor

Hygge encompasses the five senses, and food should not be left out. Drinks that are warm like coffee, tea and the glogg (Scandinavian the drink of mulled wine) as well as hearty meals such as cakes, pastries and porridge, any type of comfort food can assist you in achieving the perfect feeling of the hygge. Additionally, it's about the notion of community. food and drinks will always taste better when shared with friends.

Eight wonderful and welcoming Dens will make you be tempted to snuggle on

In the wake of the cold conditions, we're longing for an area where we can relax and be at ease. A place to cozy up with blankets, lounge before a warm fire (or an ember) or sip a hot teacup and lose ourselves in an excellent book. This is where you can discover the most warm Danes which offer exactly this, providing warm and inviting places to which we'd want to escape to during the winter cold.

Wood that has been treated with heat

The space is warm and inviting thanks to the walls thanks to the beautiful wooden panels and the crown molding that is shaped. In combination with comfortable furniture in diverse textures, including linen, leather and natural fiber carpets -

this is a space where we can look in the past.

Design tip: Use an ottoman made of leather that is larger than you need to create a sense of stability in the room. It can also serve be multi-functional for your space. It could serve as an ottoman for your feet, a coffee table, and even extra seating.

Exaggerated charm

This room demonstrates that an enthralling palette, variety of patterns and furniture from the past are still cozy and easy to move around. The heat can come in many shapes, and in this instance being able to feel that the space is bursting with an array of prints and motifs creates a more intimate atmosphere.

Design tip: A compact color palette, concentrated on red and teal and keeps the different designs and forms in check and stops the room from becoming too chaotic and unfocused.

Moody and minimalist

The dark lacquered walls transform the small room into a sanctuary for those who love of minimalist design, and serve as the main focal feature of the room, despite the absence of ornaments. It's a darker and less spacious view in the spacious jewelry area, that tends to be vibrant and more vivid walls that are brimming with ornaments.

Tips for designing: In an area that has minimal decor accents will be worn down by the elements and weather, like an old rug. A wooden coffee table adds the authentic character.

Clean elegance

Incorporating the look of an edgy Moroccan tent and a crisp traditional glaze, this room is an absolute dream, with a comfortable space to lounge and escape the cold winter chills. A neutral color palette with various shades offers the space a generous amount of warmth.

Design tip: opt for an extra-large couch bed over a couch or a set of chairs. It's an elegant upgrade, ideal for laying down and relaxing.

Texture that is neutral and rich

Bricks exposed, a crackling fireplace or a leather rug is there something in this space that can make you feel uncomfortable? Although the majority of it is brown, this room gains the richness and depth of the mix of old-fashioned materials like fur, velvet and vintage silver. It also has leather with a lovely patina.

Design tip: To create an personal and intimate atmosphere take the brick exposed as a white walls, and make a gallery using the artworks you have created as well as your personal favorites.

Nostalgia collection

Warm hues and a variety of ephemerals from the past give this place a cozy feel. We like the variety of vintage textiles, like the macrame throw as well as the Scottish pillow, which provide an extra layer of familiarity and character. The library isn't even that small (Hardy Boys, and Nancy Drew anyone?).

Design tip: Create the casual, American feel of the lake house by hanging artwork inspired by nature and gaining access to pieces that evoke nostalgia such as a ship inside bottles or an old-fashioned reading lamp.

The antiques that have been polished such as the patchwork bergere as well as the vast selection of South American art, can remain warm and inviting when you pair them with the right furniture. A comfortable seating sofa (complete by goose-down pillows) Swivel armchairs and of course the fireplace gives the atmosphere of antique treasures an aura of accessibility , making this a perfect spot to relax.

A single wall painted can add warmth and color to a space. The co-ordinated sheets make sure that it is perfectly incorporated to the surrounding space.

Cabin-Chic

From the walls and ceilings of logs to lush gardens the den may be the most luxurious cabin in the woods we've seen. Intimacy is everywhere in the combination of materials, including velvet, diamond-patterned rugs and leather as well as sheepskin (which is perfectly placed to allow feet to sink).

Design tip: In an area that has many different materials and textures, you must be precise in deciding where to apply the color by injecting it into one particular place to keep an equilibrium and polishing.

Chapter 7: How to Include a touch of Hygge in Your Everyday Routine

Cup Of Happiness

If coffee or tea are an element of your daily routine make a point to take it in completely. Incorporate a different flavor, such as cinnamon or turmeric to enhance the flavor and benefits, go for it, and then taste.

Magnificence Routine

As you go about your everyday cosmetics or skincare, try to use products that contain some calming ingredients or enjoyable material experiences to start your day. In certain instances, a facial massage is all you need to relax before starting your day.

Have Breakfast

Don't just grab the protein bar out of the front door! In the event that you have the chance for a meal with your familymembers, S.O., or even your flatmates in the beginning during the working day. It will improve your state of mind prior to starting your day.

Improve Your Workspace

Everyone doesn't need to work in an office that has zero character! Add things that make you feel and help keep the office looking beautiful and comfortable.

Take A Sip

The main element of hygge is its focus on making connections and making great memories with friends. If your friend or a friend is welcoming you to a party take it all off the table and enjoy the company of a drink or two!

Head Outside

When the temperatures are not yet a bit warm try to spend the most time outside in the time you're able. The fresh air outside can typically benefit you.

Light A Fire

Are you living with a chimney in your house? Snuggling in front of the fireplace is unique when compared with other winter hygge-related activities you could do.

Find A Scent

Candles are an additional way to make your space more comfortable. Find a scent that brings you joy and then light it when you relax.

Get cooking

Making a meal in addition to ordering take-out from a restaurant is definitely a great activity to enjoy hygge. Apart from the fact that you will enjoy the process of cooking your meals, it's a fantastic opportunity to talk with your friends from the flat or S.O. about their day.

Assemble Round

Bring your family together or invite friends over to enjoy your living space. Make sure you have comfortable elements like hide-tosses and comfy loveseats to help everyone by relaxing.

Clean up

While showers are effective they are also luxurious. If you own a tub you can take a few minutes to enjoy yourself and make the pleasure of a bath.

Relax

Prior to going to bed, ensure that you set aside a little bit of effort to relax in a comfy place.

Diary Away

Journaling can be a great way to organize your thoughts following an otherwise dull day.

Do some reading

If you're addicted to Netflix is always awe-inspiring It's an excellent idea to avoid screen time before going to going to bed.

Relax with a good book before slaying the lights.

Plan For Escapes

When you are putting aside time to improve your daily routine is remarkable, you must keep track of your plans to move with those you cherish the most.

How to Design a Hygge Bathroom

A Hygge that is fueled by inside is possible if your bathroom is clean and tidy. Maintaining your towels and toiletries at a sufficient size will help keep the mess in your bathroom in check. Vertically stockpiling your toiletries is an excellent way to reduce the space in your bathroom. It is also possible to keep stool that can be used as a location to showcase your most essentials such as books, plants, the most beloved books and candles.

The slim stockpiling cabinet is also known as a dresser, is ideal in finding clever ways to incorporate stockpiling into the space in which floor space is limited. It is ideal for space in the bathroom for stockpiling, a niche in an entrance or landing area, or as a pinnacle for stationary items for a home office.

State of Mind Light

Lighting is one of one of the easiest ways to create a warm and inviting atmosphere in the bathroom. For instance, dimmable lighting can be an excellent choice for your bathroom since it provides you with lots of light whenever you require it to create a tranquil atmosphere in the evening when you want to relax. Candles that smell good will also help you create an atmosphere of peace.

Playing with Textures

Surfaces are able to play an important role in creating the Hygge lively Bathroom. Consider mixing surfaces to give a divider to create textures that transform a cold bathroom into a comfortable one in a matter of. It is possible to settle for dense, delicate textures while selecting shower tangles, towels and even bathrobes.

Relaxing in a luxuriously soft towel and luxurious robe after an unwinding shower is what Hygge is all about.

Hygge = The concept of less is more

In terms of Hygge bathroom design We are talking about tinkering the style down. Bathrooms are typically the smallest room in your home, and in the event you must design them in an effort to create a modest style, try to be precise when choosing which space to use.

Interiors that are infused with hygge are generally easy and perfect. Selecting furniture that is moderate could be the most effective way to create the perfect bathroom hygge, starting from storage containers to mirrors. Mirrors are a must in every space. In bathrooms they aid us to prepare. In addition, in every room, they flick the lighting. A modest mirror can amplify the space.

Best Hygge Gifts For Your Coziest Winter

You're probably thinking on what's Hygge and what it possibly mean? The hottest new pattern is probably the most beautiful pattern I've any time seen. Peruse the pattern this pattern, and I'm certain that you'll be awed.

Hygee is expressed as "hoo-ga" which is an Danish concept that conveys the feeling of content, cozy, and a sense of enjoyment of the essential things in daily life. Hygee isn't more well-known and I told you how amazing it is! Absolutely my friend certainly. And who would not love a gift that makes it easier to be snug?

We picked gifts that fit right into their Hygge lifestyle and maintain in any case, at least a 4-star rating. The prices and inventory may fluctuate dependent on the time of the year.

1. Smoko Toasty Plushie Heatable

What's the difference between Netflix and chill? Slowly becoming a fan of Hulu and snuggle. Make a scene with your new friend and potato-framing the mistake of this rich friend. Let the inside of the pocket microwavable warmth you up and fill your home with the soothing scent of lavender. Also available in heart and a sloth, there are there are a variety of options.

2. The Softies ultra soft Marshmallow Hooded Luggage

The marshmallow-delicate nightwear, or, as I like to refer to them Self-Care Sunday Fashion was included on The Oprah Show's Favorite Things List for 2019. What if she said she's ever been off base on what she is talking about? The short answer is probably not. In addition, how do be honest, if it's enough for Oprah then it's sufficient for you.

3. Delicious Insane Sweets

If the thought of heating up a few amazing yummy Death by Chocolate brownies (that's correct, it's an original recipe) will feel hygge-like and you're there, imagine how relaxed you'll feel as you breathe in the entire scrumptiousness of your baked desserts. Additionally, with 100 plans, you'll never get exhausted--regardless of whether your appliance's staying at work past 40 hours all winter.

4. Avocado-Holic Socks

Imagine toasting avocados (or even better by having your companion make toast for you) dressed in these adorable socks. Furthermore, as they're made of a fine cotton blend, and have a cushioned comfort sole they're on the same level as the style.

5. My Sheets are rock "The Normal" Sheets

They're made from the best bamboo fabric These sheets aren't just fragile as margarine (and become more gentle after each washing!). But they also control the temperature and absorb dampness (read you won't sweat on your mattress when you're snoozing beneath your down-quill bed).

Additionally, they're quite inexpensive, which makes them the perfect present to offer yourself. Oh, and did I note that this fitted sheet comes with the corner with a label that tell you exactly what corner to place it on. This is self-care.

6. Shower Bombs for Bubbles, Bubbles Donuts

These shower bombs with a cake flavor can make a relaxing shower while reading an ebook or watching your favorite TV show, in fact, significantly better (quip that is completely expected). If the floral and fruity scent doesn't convince you, then at this time, perhaps a lady named Ellen Degeneres will. They're listed on her list of her most beloved things. Doughnut attempts to create Hygge without the need for.

7. Cozy Coloring Book

Hygge isn't just about watching your favorite shows, but rather being wrapped all around in soft, comfortable fabrics. It could be mostly about that, but it is also connected to using your imagination muscles, if you're aware, that's the factor that relaxes your muscles.

The book's cozy shade will be a good choice for "what could be like an uninteresting cover" which means you'll have confidence when unwinding (regardless of whether you'll take some time to talk the pencils using a purple- or burgundy-hued).

Say what you want about Uggs okay Fine, they're essential fashion. But, it is impossible to ignore the simple pleasure that is flowing through these extremely cozy, terrible young men. Shoes? They're becoming increasingly like tiny mists on your feet.

This pair of socks (accessible in dark, charcoal cream, and dark) is a warm shearling fleece that joins with a soft sew. Find a place on the rack for shoes since you'll be wearing these throughout the winter long.

9. Quality Blankets with Weighted Fillings

Oh, the weighted cover, a.k.a. the current trend in wellness that fights for the right cause. With proven benefits such as helping relax you and ease your mind this promotion is sure to be a hit. There's also no better time on a chilly winter night to join involved in the weighted-cover temporary trend.

Comfortable, cozy and with the ability to give you the feeling that you're being loved, this cover with five stars from Amazon is an ideal way to relax in frigid temperatures. More than 8,000 commentators aren't correct.

10. We Are Knitters Kilim Blanket Knitting Kit

If covers that weigh 20 pounds aren't your thing then why not make your own and sit by the fireplace (or space heater) for the entire winter? This DIY kit by We Is Knitters will show how to make an ideal cover that is separate from others. (No to be a fake, just genuine.) Best part? There's a second Hygge blessing once you're done!

Ideas for gifts for the Hygge Lover

These beautiful notecards from Kinfolk are a fantastic choice for small presents. The Hygge Edition is a perfect representation of the cosy tradition of hygge and it truly is a gift that keeps giving since it is used to share love long after the present has been accepted. The Hygge Edition is packaged in a high-quality wooden box contains twelve collapsible cards of A2 size with vibrant interiors and full-shading spreads of photography and twelve envelopes that are clear.

For a hygge or shut-in lover, it is impossible to be too stuffed with candles.

On the chance that you're not sure what to gift someone it is always a good idea because it's valuable. The tall, beautiful candles through Hygge Life are engraved with the well-known Royal Copenhagen flatware structure with environmentally friendly ink. The colors are dark, red great blue, and dark.

If you've got a friend who needs to be energized or perhaps a family member who's feeling slightly sick or has relocated to a new home, this personalized blessing box on Etsy is an amazing gift that you can send directly to the recipient and brighten up their day. The case is secured by a band that is printed with a beautiful paper-like plan (the kind of material that the most beautiful covers are created with) with the suggestion that staying at home, in the middle. Inside, you'll find an overview of the contents and a recommendation to light a fire and snuggle in a warm or a calming hug, spend time with loved ones and enjoy the simple things that happen in daily life.' Great!

Who doesn't adore a Hygge scented room diffuser? This one is from Skandinavisk available from Skandium is reminiscent of blended tea , flowers, strawberry cakes as well as wild mint. It is a scent that will last for at least three months, and will provide an ideal atmosphere for those who aren't used to the most regular minutes.

I am in love with this cute cushion featuring the print 'Hyggekrog An alcove for you to snuggle in, relax and relax. Bring the feeling of hygge into the home of someone you love with this cozy Hygge quotes pad. The faux cowhide texture makes this pad luxurious on the touch and gorgeous to snuggle up with.

In the event that the person you're buying as a gift loves tea, then it is a good idea to purchase one of the tasty teas of Hoogly Tea is excellent! Isn't there something to be said about Danish Pastry, a free leaf tea? It has a deliciously warm scent of cinnamon and chocolate, and an unassumingly delicious baked good-taste the sound of this guilty delight is sure to entice tea lovers repeatedly.

These comfy, nervy cashmere-fleece mix socks are amazing ideas for all. Perfect for relaxing and reminding your pals or family members to bring you the best thing to spend a relaxing, hygge-inspired moment with your family or friends wine! It is made from QineThree to Hygge North, and is available in three distinctive shades navy force, dark or dim.

A stunning little reminder of the importance of taking advantage of the essential pleasures: a charming vintage spoon that has 'hygge' engraved on the inside accessible on Etsy. This means that every you have a cup of coffee or tea, they'll think of the word hygge. Each piece is individually stepped each letter by hand and the flatware is a vintage silver-plated.

Do you have a loved one who loves the normal life? This mug in the shape of a sloth comes from Urban Outfitters will be an amazing little friend and will always bring a smile to their faces. Look at the expression on his face! I think I'm in need of one.

A small, thoughtful, and useful blessing is this schedule stickers by Grand Stories Design - for anyone who loves Hygge. The pack includes 70 labels. Make use of these for exceptional day-to-day stamping, focus on the important things and let them awaken to add a touch of warmth to your daily. You can use it as a calendar or to decorate a card you're giving to your friend.

For someone who is a shut-in such as me, a great idea (and something that the person might not yet have) is to create a guestbook. Every thing that happens at your home, each time you have a gathering, and the simple coffees that are a loyal friend - all leave an footprints. This guestbook by Ferm Living offers a prestigious experience from every single moment of it, which will remain even after the party is over. It showcases the pages of 192 pages that are a masterpiece of paper, silk strip, as well as a distinctive high-quality art using metallic gold on the hardcover.

Chapter 8: Appreciating the Everyday Moments

The pace of life is so busy that we can take our eyes off of the world around us. We are unable to see the small actions that could provide us with tiny moments of joy. Such as that smile from the clerk at the grocery store or the kind gesture of the person who waited patiently for you in the elevator.

Our focus is solely focused on ourselves and the things we must do throughout the day, and we aren't paying attention to the objects or people that are around us. It is essential to relax and allow space for the small things in our lives.

To take note of the small things in life to appreciate the small things, first you need to recognize factors that keep us smile.

Pause and think about how to identify your things you're grateful for. To determine the small things you're grateful for, ask yourself a question.

What are the most obvious things you'd be missing If they weren't there?

What makes me feel content in my everyday life?

What are the things that make me feel happy every day?

Example:

The morning cup of coffee helps you to be more alert.

You can watch a film in the comfort of your sofa with your loved one.

A telephone call you make to your most loved friend or mother.

You are listening to your favorite tune while you commute to work.

Make sure to buy things that are inexpensive or free in comparison to the material items. The satisfaction you get from purchasing goods that aren't worth the cost is a short. If however you are satisfied to have an item of clothing because it brings back an event that you were happy about and you are happy, then it could be included on your list of reasons to be feel grateful.

There are plenty of things that bring you joy every day You just need to look for them.

This list will grow longer and longer as time passes as you become more aware of the tiny events in your life.

The next morning, you can enjoy your cup of coffee with more focus so that happiness is able to flow through you.

Through these small exercises, you'll be aware of people and things who can make you feel happier.

When you're more conscious of your daily routine, you'll notice what you're missing.

Begin to pay attention to the internal organs and outside. Perhaps you'd like to exercise more. Make a place to train in the gym, or take a stroll or whatever is what makes you feel happy.

It is likely that you won't get it right the first time you attempt it, but trying new experiences can make you feel more present. The excitement you feel when you try something new can definitely enhance your life.

You could revisit the old passion. Something you enjoyed doing back in the past, but that you've not been able to do anymore due to the fact that you've learned away from other pursuits. It could be a game that you participated in as a child or a hobby you enjoyed when you were a kid, such as writing or painting. Take a notebook or a canvas, lie in a chair and begin creating or writing.

You'll see that the things you used to love are now your favorites.

Split your time in different ways

The day-to-day life of the majority of people is arranged in this way:

Dress yourself, wake up get ready for work, lunch, home, work dinner, television then go to bed and get ready for the next day.

In this way, we're no longer in charge of our lives. The daily routine of our lives is planned. We are only able to determine the time between the phases. We're like tram drivers. The stops have been made. You can only accelerate or slow down.

We often make excuses that our day is too short for other things. In reality, this isn't an excuse. It simply indicates that we can't split our time efficiently.

What would be the experience If I switched the location for my lunch break? You could take your own food from home , or take your lunch break in the park.

Do you think your coworkers may think that you are a bit sexist?

It's normal, but the smile on your face when you are looking at your food could make your friends look jealous.

In that moment you have broken a custom or a norm, something that most others aren't able to.

In the evening, following dinner, rather than sitting watching the television and watching the news, sip the glass of your preferred wine while listening to your preferred music.

You can also go through a book you placed on the shelves and made yourself promise to take the time to read.

You're more productive than you think you do and don't let it be consumed by the dull moments of your day such as a day at work.

Create a list of things which consume a large amount or all of your attention. Most likely, the time you spend on social media is enough to scare you.

Set your phone down and consider what would truly make you feel happy.

Smartphones - the cause of unhappy

The smartphone is certainly an amazing invention that allows us to keep connected to our loved ones as well as keep up to date with the latest news.

A lot of use on the phone can cause the opposite result, i.e. unhappiness. It is because we need to be in the forefront of things and stay informed of everything.

A study conducted by scientists has shown that viewing images on social media could cause you to feel unhappy, or even depressed.

You can do an experiment. Download a free App (there are a variety of) which calculates the amount of the time that you are spending on social networking, the amount you make use of your smartphone as well as how many times it is necessary to unlock the phone, and more. You'll find that this information is unimaginable for you. If you now know how much time you're spending using your phone and the amount of time it is stealing from your life, you can take steps to cut down on its usage.

It is common for us to use our smartphones to get around time. When we stand in line at the grocery store or while waiting to see the physician during commercials on TV or when waiting for food that we have ordered at the restaurant to be delivered the possibilities are infinite.

If you attempt to use your phone more, you'll be able for other activities.

In the beginning, it may be difficult to adjust to it. You should also be careful not to answer your phone.

Here is a list of possibilities for you to do:

Contact a friend via the phone

Check out old photos

A novel read

Listen to the music

Read an issue of a magazine

Set your schedule for the week ahead

Planning an excursion

Take a stroll

A friend you've not seen in a long time

Cook a tasty food

Reviving an old pastime

Awestruck by the beauty of the scenery and becoming enthralled by thoughts

The list of tasks is long but this is just one small portion.

Doing any of the activities listed or any other thing that occurs to your mind, can give you more emotion than just focusing using your phone.

Make Hygge a part of your life with other people

Once you've been able to put down your phone and catch up with the things you love doing, you can feel a sense of hygge who are around you. Your family or your friends.

Sharing laughter and conversation with friends and family members is vital to creating a sense of Hygge. Being together makes us feel less lonely and social interactions can make us feel more joyful. The act of sharing and discussing news is about being with others. The stress of worry is also an aspect of being in a relationship Sharing the concerns we have with our loved ones helps us to overcome our fears and defeat them.

Going to the movies and chatting on the film or having a cup of coffee at a new café or perhaps playing board games with your buddies are all things that can make you feel more connected and enhance your Hygge.

The most effective way to increase your hygge is to share meals and drinks with your family and friends.

The table is always a fun and convivial gathering place for family and acquaintances. A meal shared with your loved ones , or sipping glasses of wine or coffee can make everyone more social. The food can be large or sweet. A delicious roast that is accompanied by grilled veggies as well as a refreshing glasses of red wine. When you consume all of them together it makes the food taste better.

The Danes especially love desserts, as do all Scandinavians. Sweets aid the Danes to survive the winter months and shield against depression. This isn't to be overlooked due to the absence of sunlight.

A relaxing afternoon spent with friends with tea, coffee or hot chocolate is extremely cozy.

Food is a fantastic occasion to enhance your hygge. Make a point of preparing your meals, and take pleasure in each bite mindfully.

How do you stay Hygge

Hygge is effective on cold and hot days. Hygge can be enjoyed all year long. In winter the walls are warm and inviting, and in summer, outdoor activities are the most popular.

Below we outline what things to do to ensure that each season is cozy as you can.

Autumn

The days are becoming shorter. The sun is getting less, and the nature is coloured by warm hues. It's a great moment to take in nature as well as for relaxing evenings:

Relaxing on the couch and reading the latest book.

Prepare your winter garden.

A relaxing bath after a long, cold winter.

Go for a stroll in the woods to pick chestnuts , or just listen to nature and take a whiff of the wood.

Make a hot soup and make it available to the rest of your friends.

Pause during a rainy day and listen to the sounds of rain.

Winter

It is the darkest and coldest season, but that doesn't mean that you need to lower your temperature. This is the time when the Hygge takes over the house.

Cooking up hot meals to serve family and friends.

Make a warm and cozy ambience with candles.

Enjoying the first snowfall.

How to make snowmen.

Enjoy your music and pay more focus on the parts of songs you didn't notice and that bring you powerful emotions.

Go to the Christmas markets.

Find Christmas presents to give away and pack them.

Decorate your Christmas home.

Enjoy a stroll and feel the cool breeze that swathes your face.

Spring

"Open the windows and let the sun's new light, which is spring." He was singing a tune. The landscape changes and turns brighter. Green is the color of most dominant, but there are also red, yellow, and white. The sunshine rays make us feel more comfortable and the days are getting longer.

There are a variety of activities you can take part in outdoors during this time.

A bicycle ride to meet up with friends in the bar.

Utilizing the bike to get to work.

Find flowers in the fields and place these in an arrangement to bring your home a fresh spring air.

Take care of your home after a winter that has been long. A tidy home is an ideal way to bring your spirits back to.

Place your flowers in the garden , or in vases that add scent and color to your everyday surroundings.

Markets are where you can find bargains such as books, old books, and old records.

Summer

The days are becoming longer and warmer. There's enough time take in the sun and the natural world.

Plan a barbecue party with your people you know that continues until late in the evening.

Plan trips. It is not necessary to travel far to feel disengaged. Even short weekends can make you feel better.

A picnic with your friends.

Take in the beautiful sunset while you sip a bottle of vino.

Go to the ocean

Garden care

Be sure to enjoy the stars at night.

Relax on the beach next to the fire and discuss some other stories.

Chapter 9: Hygge And The Art Of Being Together

"Harmony": This isn't just a contest. We already have a great relationship with you. It is not necessary to boast about your accomplishments."

The appeal of hygge lies in its being an inexplicably concept. It's not a concept that can be explained in only a few experiences. One of the greatest features of hygge parties or the Danish style of living is that they do not feel to be a burden or attract attention to themselves. It's about shedding the mask of self-consciousness, being authentic and having meaningful conversations while also enhancing the sense of belonging. Cultural bonds, social ties small rituals of community and receiving assistance from family members are woven in the Danish lifestyle.

How can people gather and create a hygge atmosphere to beat stress and create strong bonds of friendship. This is everything you need to be aware of about social hygge.

1. Stay Drama-Free

Danish social gatherings or hygges aren't teeming with tension, debates that are controversial and competition. There's absolutely no room for displaying pride. There aren't any negative remarks on people, slanderous gossip or complains about how life is a mess. The air is filled with positive energy, and there's no room for negative comments. People don't boast about their accomplishments or challenge one another (so which vehicle model is the most up-to-date?).

There's an unspoken rule that restricts conversations to subjects that allow people to enjoy the company of their family members.

It's a bit strange for people who aren't and yet hygge is so much of an obsession in Danish society that it's gradually entering their workplaces too. As a person from a different culture You'll be amazed by how Danes have their professional colleagues by creating a relaxing ambience with dim lighting as well as fragrant candles and comfy seating in conference rooms.

Don't be surprised by the fact that your Danish business partner gives you a huge cushion to sit on in a crucial business meeting. The reason is that it's an ode to the renowned and joyful Danish culture. They don't do it to promote their own culture , but simply because that's how they are. People who seek comfort, happiness and ever giving. There is a greater focus on creating an environment that is familiarity, connectivity and ease than on tension.

2. All things are teamwork

Making the effort to make the task more enjoyable for everyone is crucial to the concept of social hygge. As with other societies, everyone aims to be productive and involved. Social hygges are lovely and meaningful as everyone contributes to the preparation of meals, serving them and then cleaning them up.

In contrast to other cultures, it's is not just the host who has an errand at the kitchen table serving guests, but also wishing they could be spending more time with guests. Everyone is involved and socializing with others, making meals and having enjoyable. The Hygge spirit doesn't revolve around one person working out, while everyone else is enjoying themselves. It's about sharing and conversing and creating a naturally communal feeling over shared activities and meals.

What makes these social hygges so attractive are the simple fact Danes do not like to over complicate things like planning the menu and so on. They prefer to keep things easy so that they are able to spend more time engaging with other people. You'll not have an elaborate meal on the evenings of hygge. It's home-cooked and served with boiling soup. It will also be an easy such as roasting chicken. They prefer simple and tasty food without extras.

3. Get the most out of your Time

The Danes are awestruck by even the tiniest of moments of community and are more conscious of their surroundings because they know that their time here on earth and with one another is short. Hygges are about staying present in the moment and savoring the beauty of it by prolonging the moment.

It's not just about filling up your mouth with food, and then moving off to another gathering. It's about taking time to enjoy each bite and taking time to linger over food, and engaging with laughter and conversation. It's about creating lasting memories with food.

They turn off everything else like the phone or television, and focus on having fun with their family and friends with food and drinks.

4. Let Get Rid from the outside World

One of the basic unspoken rules that is the basis of Danish"social hygge" is that you let the world go when you go into someone's sanctuary. It's about enjoying the safety of your loved ones and family's company.

The outdoor temperatures can be chilly and bitter in winter This is the reason why many seek refuge in the company of their loved ones inside. This is not the place to debate office politics or boast about your new job. It's a place where people can have amusement, spill their hearts out to each other and be in touch, without room for anyone to judge one another. In a hygge that is social, Individuals don't have to be concerned about being judged, or being viewed as less than.

The best way to demolish the hygge effect is to brag about your achievements. The Danes rarely talk about their accomplishments or achievements. They often minimize their achievements in order for others to feel happy about their own achievements. That's how the hygge environment operates.

In reality, a Hygge is a way to escape the world of competitiveness outside in which everyone is striving to be better than the one another at a rapid speed. It is not a good idea to bring the same competitive streak into a the hygge. This is due to the socially inclusive Scandinavian culture, in which any notion of superiority is considered to be a sin.

Be sure to keep your eyes off distractions including devices and smartphones, especially when dining. Because hygge is about creating the feeling of being connected to your loved ones, and experiencing the joy of being in their presence, technology is massive hygge-related spoilers.

Hygge could be described as an ideal alternative to the contemporary lifestyle. It's all about taking in the moment, which can be difficult as we constantly stare at our phones and trying to create virtual connections that are not real important bonds. Put down your phone and listening to the conversations of others goes in the spirit of hygge. Enjoy the experience of being with your beloved ones and take advantage of your time spent with them.

There is nothing as unhygge-like as politics because everything that is controversial is automatically excluded from the notion of Hygge. Hygge is more traditional, traditional and communal events and are meant to be relaxed and casual. Danish is a society that views Hygge as a method of hiding your power.

It demands that you be part of the world regardless of what position you have in society. Hygge is considered to be a sanctuary where you can put aside all names and social distinctions to relax and enjoy games, food conversations, and the company of your loved ones. It's an escape, a way to stay away from the world while enjoying special moments with those who matter.

The importance of highlighting differences is a key part of the concept of social hygge. Denmark is a largely agricultural state, and the people were closely connected with the growing crop, even though the country was developing quickly. The adherence to traditional culture and tradition was crucial to maintain their traditional lifestyle in the midst of the rapid growth. Hygge is a source of harmony and accord. Dissent or rebellion doesn't make much sense in Danish lifestyle. Everyone must be at ease, cozy and content.

5. The Hygge Food

As we've mentioned earlier food is an integral part of the hygge lifestyle of sharing as well as bonding and comfort in the company of others. It's not about making food an extravagant, seven-course event, but rather making it simple, home-cooked and delicious. It's all about serving, cooking and sharing meals in a cozy and welcoming setting. Freshly baked bread and desserts are the most essential part of Danish Hygge. People gather together and invest their souls and hearts into the simple task making bread.

Hygges are a great source of warm drinks and comfort food to provide a cozy ambience. The majority of Danish establishments create a cozy ambience at sunset (thinks many beautiful candles, a back fireplace), Danish hygges are not about emptying your pockets or spending a lot of money. They're about seeking coziness as well as connection and comfort.

There are freshly baked cakes as well as open-faced sandwiches meatballs, roast chicken and unlimited cups of coffee hot in traditional Danish Hygges. For North America, it will be more about hot chocolate as well as chicken pot recipes and baking chocolate-y cakes.

The smoky aroma of freshly baked bread of bread wafting through the house is as cozy as it could be. The dough is carefully and cathartically made, and then you can enjoy freshly baked bread while spending time with family and friends is one of the most simple, yet most precious joys.

A popular hygge tradition is serving guests a hot cup of cocoa that is slowly stirred over the stove, using authentic chocolate, milk as well as thick, creamy cream. The rich, fine chocolatey mixture is served in large mugs and distributed in a cozy environment, while you chat with your friends and family. Delicious bliss!

Hygge is all about taking pleasure with the wonderful things in life that make you smile (read cakes and pastries). It's all about making yourself satisfied and not being in a state of deprivation from these simple pleasures.

Hygge food is a synonym for joy clearly and loudly. You don't have to sacrifice calories or savory goodness. This isn't as much about professionalism or perfectionism for the Danes but rather the love that goes into the act of creating food that is fresh. Traditional and traditional cuisines are preferred over modern fast food.

The fun is in creating the food with your family and friends in a truly rural setting, complete with a fireplace and various natural elements of the outdoors brought indoors. The best way to maximize the spirit of hygge is inviting everyone cooking in a group, not just one person being the host.

The most important investment that Danes make is a cozy and sturdy wooden dining table that is able to seat with a few people. Since a large portion of their happiness revolves around food with their loved family members, they place an emphasis on the design of the ideal dining table.

Sharing one's home with guests is a common and normal thing that is commonplace in Danish society. It's all about creating the perfect dining experience with candles lit, filling the glasses and making the food easy. An excessive fuss over food and stressing over taking too long cooking can dampen the spirit of hygge which the Danes are well aware of.

If you'd like to entertain like the Danes and have a great time, it's all about sticking with basic tasty, yet delicious, snacks and sweets as you sit down to enjoy a great time with your guests. Make sure that the schnapps and beverages are flowing and everyone is happy. Danes love to host for hours and stay after dinner to enjoy activities. The game of charades, or Scrabble perhaps?

Marie Tourell Soderberg, author of Hygge: The Danish Art of Happiness, suggests making Snorbrod (a sweet version of marshmallow roasting to make Smores) to create an ideal hygge. Nothing is more cozy than wrapping dough around sticks and baking it over an open flame to brown. It's a source of stimulating for all senses like sensing the smell of the fire and watching the flames roar as they roar, and feeling the warmness to your own body.

A truly Nordic gathering isn't complete without eating an open-faced sandwich, commonly known as smorrebrod Denmark. It's as simple and flexible as you can get yet still an excellent comfort food. Add a variety of ingredients with no frills and don't require heat to serve buffet style. Place the table in a place by baking fresh rye bread, and various spreads. You can also top it off with fresh vegetables.

Make creative pairings of spreads and veggies, such as the fresh spread of carrots that is paired with salted salmon. It is easy to arrange everything on the table so that guests are able to assist themselves and build their own sandwiches. Make a lettuce base and then add other ingredients like egg slices, fresh vegetables, mustard and various types of cheese. The guests of the party can freely communicate with each other as they make their own food and enjoying the company of their family members.

Porridge isn't just another comfort food within the Danish food culture. It's a method of gathering people over breakfast or family meals. Create a large bowl of oatsand and add flavor by adding apple and spices (cinnamon) and other delicious toppings. The whole dish is nutritious and delicious. It's a fusion of warmth and comfort, which is essential to the essence of Hygge. Making healthy, simple and trimmed-free meals is the essence of hygge.

6. Christmas Hygge

The Christmas hygge phenomenon is a huge deal when Danes also have their own name for it, namely julehygge or Christmas Hygge. Although there's no stopping hygge throughout the year as a cultural obsession however, they are at their peak at the season of Christmas. Hygge becomes the focal point for a whole month of celebrations, festivities as well as social events.

Danish Christmas celebrations almost always be centered around the hygge concept, even though the festivities aren't too different from what they do in other western countries.

We've all heard about Denmark's love affair with light. From fairy lights to costly candles to beautiful lampshades, light shows come to life in all shapes in the Danish Christmas season, with its brightly lit celebrations. According to research carried out by the Happiness Research Institute, 28 percent of the Danish population light candles on a daily basis while 85 percent identify hygge to burning candles. This is because candles are a part of the Danish notion of hygge.

Meik Wiking, the CEO of Copenhagen's Happiness Research Institute, talks about an ordinary Christmas Day story, spent with a tight-knit group of members in a cozy wooden cabin. After a very exhausting snow trek, the friends are seated around a fire, sporting sweaters and wool socks and listened to the flames of the fireplace roar up, and sipping an ice-cold glass. One of the people present asked "Could it be any more cozy?" Everyone nodded in unison as another said, "Yes, if a storm was to rage outside." This sums up the essence of hygge. The idea of creating a cozy haven and a sense of comfort when the conditions are difficult to venture out.

Relaxing at home and reflect is part of Denmark's collective mind. Contrary to Americans and the American way of thinking that being busy is a sign of being important is not present in the psyche. Finally, we have time to take to read, draw and write.

7. Winter Hygge Gatherings

Social gatherings in winter are usually held at home or in comfortable bars, cafes and eateries. The latter is all about having a meal together and spending time with family and friends. It's more of an informal evening where people can let their hair down and engage in a conversation that is fun and lighthearted. Simple, home-cooked platters of baked goods and cups of hot coffee are made rounds through the warm dimly lit living rooms. There are people drinking wine while warming themselves in front of the fireplace.

One of the best suggestions when you're trying to recreate the hygge ambience is to stick with fresh and seasonal winter food and stay clear of processed, packaged labels. The Danish prefer to make their own desserts made with fresh ingredients available. Simple and natural is the premise of the concept of hygge Remember? You can incorporate food items that are available especially during winter.

The winter hygge parties are held at cozy cafes and bars, community clubs, and eateries. There are even warmly-lit antique-style cozy bookstores. Any place that is nourishing to your soul is an ideal hygge spot. You can think of making hygge enjoyable by gathering over an evening of card or board games. In certain Copenhagen restaurants "hyggers" take part in board games with complete strangers in order to make friends and spark off a conversation.

Do you want to meet strangers in your community? You can put up a notice that says "Hygge" (you'd clearly explain the meaning of hygge to those who aren't familiar with it) outside a well-known café or bar inviting people to come and mingle with each other in games or conversations. Perhaps an hygge reading group for books as well as Mexican food club Hygge? Hygge can be incorporated into any meaningful or enjoyable social event. Think knitting clubs and poker clubs, chess events, Uno clubs, and photography groups.

Hygge is all about making connections. And what better way to make connections than to hang out with like-minded people, over the same interests and sharing fun.

Winter clothing is an essential component of Hygge. The intimate, comfortable and cozy winter vibe can't be complete without cozy clothing. Clothes are viewed as a means of showing yourself affection, love and indulgence. It's all about luxury clothing, cashmere trousers, sheepskin slip-ons made of wool, sheepskin socks and much more. It's all about staying inside and embracing the hygge vibe. Don your best oversized socks, luxe leggings and cozy leggings.

8. Play

Gaming is a very hygge activity and hygge-like in Danish culture. Playing cards or playing the game of board games, or engaging in outdoor sports with friends games are a great method to bond through an exciting and healthy sport. It's about having fun and having fun in the present.

Another hygge-related activity that is fun is to sing along. Although it may sound cheesy to different cultures, it brings people and is guaranteed to keep everyone happy. A lot of families have their own tune which has significance to their lives. Every time they gather to celebrate a special event and they tend to host a large celebration, with all the games and a sing-dance routine.

Yes it is true that the Danes are able to make every meal one of a kind, especially during Christmas and Thanksgiving.

They're not a method to create a sense of superiority or one-upmanship. It's a chance to connect with your loved ones through enjoyable activities that you can share.

Chapter 10: How to Use Hygge in Your Life

People love feeling comfortable at home, content, and serene And you do not need to relocate to Denmark in order to live a Hygge-like lifestyle. There are many ways to incorporate aspects of Hygge into your home and daily life. If you incorporate these principles into your daily life you will be able to bring out feelings of harmony, comfort and tranquility in your daily life.

Lighting

It is essential to upgrade your lighting if you are looking to incorporate elements in the style of Hygge in your home. A soft , warm white light creates an atmosphere that is comfortable and welcoming in comparison to stark and bright white bulbs. The bulbs will shine more bright if it has more lumens. You can put in an dimmer to keep track of the lighting of the room that you reside in. Another thing to consider is having floor lamps rather than overhead lighting. They will produce lighting that is way too intense for the space. It could make the room look a bit formal. When you make use of floor and table lamps, it can be a great way to create a space that feels intimate by using the most effective lighting. Also, make sure that you illuminate the areas where people sit and relax and talk to one another or read. Candles are the most enjoyable aspect of living a more hyggelig style. They provide a warm and soft lighting that leaves you feeling peace and comfort. If an open-flamed candle poses danger for your home due to pets or children You can opt for LED lighting.

Texture

Hygge is the term used to describe objects that are cozy and comfortable. Include accessories like pillows and blankets, rug and throws to make your space comfortable and cozy. Soft textures can

127

help soothe you, especially when anxiety is running high. Soft textures can also help you to provide people with a assurance. Decorating your living space can allow people to connect with one another. Conversations with others will be more relaxed and open within this space. No one will feel pressured or stressed.

Decor

It is possible to create a peaceful atmosphere by adding different items such as indoor plants, wood pieces and minimalist decoration. It is recommended to use these items in particular, particularly those with an important meaning. It is possible to keep photos of your family, friends and other beloved ones in the fireplace of your living space. You could also put some books on the coffee table, with photos of your adventures and trips that you might have shared with people who are around you. Hygge is all about connection and warmth, therefore you must use the design to attract your family and friends into your home, and to spark conversations.

Warmth

It is essential to realize that warmth doesn't only about the temperature of the room it also includes a feeling emotion-based warmth. One of the most effective ways to live a more hygge-like way of life is to create an open fireplace. However, this isn't an option for everyone. There are many ways to can create a warm, welcoming area, and this can be a benefit. A few examples include candles and lights, displays, accent lighting and many more. It is also possible to use twinkly lights or fairy lights in the areas around your home in order to provide warmth. These alternatives can be used to substitute for fireplaces.

Color

The color you pick for your living area can create a warm and inviting space for your friends, yourself and loved ones. It is best to select the neutral hues such as whites, soft pastel browns, whites and blushes. When you select neutral shades, you can relax the mind, and set a peaceful environment. The colors that you choose will be suitable for the Hygge style of living. The Hygge style of living is about creating a relaxing, comfortable, relaxing, or tranquil environment. In simple terms it is about creating a relaxing, comfortable, and peaceful environment. Hygge lifestyle creates the environment to be a relaxing one and allows you to spend time with people you cherish.

People

As previously mentioned as a result, the Hygge lifestyle is focused on establishing and maintaining relationships with family members. It is important to remain present. If you cultivate these connections, you allow yourself and others who surround you to feel the feeling of peace. If you're in a place where you are a part of, you'll feel safe and secure. If you are able to maintain your emotional security, you can have an enjoyable social experience. This will let you enjoy the benefits of peace connectedness, peace, and security.

Activity

A hyggelig life style will include items that help you feel comfortable at ease, comfortable, and calm. You'll learn to be able to communicate with those who surround you easily. One of the most effective ways to accomplish this is by spending time with family and friends. These gatherings focus solely on connecting with people close to you and not just about the surrounding. It is not necessary to have a formal black tie occasion. The Hygge style will suggest something different. These events will enable the opportunity to create an environment that is welcoming, relaxed and gives people an opportunity to concentrate on interacting with others in the vicinity. The atmosphere will help participants to feel at home. You can arrange an evening of games with your family members, friends or your neighbors, organize an evening of reading or invite friends to join you for a meal or coffee.

A Few Tips

Here are some tips you can follow to live an hygge-like lifestyle.

Light Candles

Wiking claims that it is impossible to adhere to the Hygge lifestyle in the absence of candles. This is stated in the very first section of his book. When you turn the light down and put candles in your home, you are able to change the ambience you're within with ease. To improve the experience you can make use of scented candles that bring peace to the space. It's impossible to not enjoy the soothing effect of the scent and the gentle glow from the burning flame. The aroma and scent is a major aspect in living the

Hygge lifestyle. If certain scents or perfumes make you think of an experience that made you feel comfortable and secure, they will remind you of Hygge.

Never Deprive Yourself

It is essential to are enjoying the little pleasures of your life. It also means that should enjoy whatever you like doing and being gentle with yourself. The Danes love sweets as well as other sweets such as gummy bears and licorice. Make sure that you don't concentrate solely on your diet and take every opportunity to indulge in the delights that you are entitled to.

Take an Hot Cup of Tea

Have you ever felt more relaxed after sipping the hot tea covered in a warm blanket? If yes, you ought to enjoy the taste of peppermint tea or any other tea that you enjoy. Wiking offers an emergency Hygge list that is tied to the pleasure to take a breather, and the Hygge idea of relaxation.

Unwind

Hygge can encourage you spending time with people you cherish. However, this doesn't mean that you must always be with people. One of the great things to be said about Hygge way of life is that one are able to relax and take time to pamper yourself. Apply a face mask and repair your skin with the most effective moisturizing formulation, or any other thing that can assist you in relaxing. You could also apply some lotion, soak in a tub or apply nail polish. It is essential to take advantage of this type of relaxation if you wish to live the Hygge way of life.

Create an Playlist

The perfect music will always create the perfect mood. When you design music that is perfect for your time with family or friends, or even an the evening alone and invite positive energy and comfort to the space. It is also possible to relax your body quickly. Install speakers and listen to your favorite music.

Bring the Outdoors inside

Danes dislike sitting in the house during winter. They like to bring the outdoors into the home. They love everything made from wood, and that includes things from nature such as twigs, nuts, plants, and so on. The aroma of the fireplace as well as other wooden items can make you feel more connected to the natural world. They are easy to use and stay true to the notion of Hygge. It is possible to find objects that embody the natural world with musky wood and other woods with textured textures.

Have a book handy

It is also essential to keep a copy of your book on hand. This is a crucial task to complete. After a longand hard day, it's better to lose yourself within the pages the book. It could be a memoir, how-to guide or your the book you have always loved. Be sure to choose the book that will put you at comfortably. Don't skim through the book as this would not be a very relaxing way to go. Allow the story to unfold and take note of where it takes you. It is important to take in everything.

Unplug

Most people find that the devices they use are their lifelines. If you shut it down, and switch off your computer even for an hour, you're doing yourself an favor. This might seem like a daunting task but it will aid you in becoming more present. It will help you become more aware of your surroundings. This is one of the most important aspects about Hygge. Hygge will allow you to tell your brain when you're away from work.

Make Your Space Cozy

Huge blankets and pillows are important. This is particularly true if you wish to convey an atmosphere warm and provide a relaxing space. You can improve the atmosphere by adding blankets and pillows. It is possible to use soothing ingredients such as chamomile, patchouli and lavender to brighten the atmosphere. These scents will give you feelings of peace and security. It is crucial to create a tranquil and secure space in order to make your home appear more cozy.

Add twinkly lights

It is a good idea to have a twinkly light at the home. Like we said earlier, lighting is one of the greatest aspects of an Hygge way of life. The lights are bright and bright and look fantastic anyplace. These lights can be placed in your living space or bedroom, or outside on your patio.

Light a fire

One of the best things about the Danish culture is the ability to gather around the flame. The fire can be outdoors or indoors. It is the ideal time to be able to spend time with family, friends and beloved ones. It is important to be grateful for the people you surround yourself with. A fireplace is a symbol of unity and warmth. It is a place where people can relax and spend time with loved ones.

Open Presents at the Right Moment

This is a notion that is found in many Hygge books. It is a crucial idea to keep in mind. It's always a great idea to purchase special packages to mark your achievements or milestones. Once you are able to appreciate these items, you'll discover how to tie every piece that you have in your home to some joyful memories.

The Planning Hygge Factors are in Every Room

If you are planning to renovate your home it is important to plan the interior decor of your space. If you were planning this, you may not pay focus on the emotional aspects of the design. Also, you didn't think about the many memories you'd be making within these rooms. Hygge can help you design the elements of each space. For instance, if you were concerned about the wallpaper in your bedroom while you were renovating your home, you wouldn't have considered the impact it could have on your morning routine or how it would affect reading in the evening. Soon, you will be able to decorate your home so that you and those you love feel more comfortable.

Chapter 11: Tips to live in harmony and be able to accommodate People with a few daily gists

Harmony with others can be quite challenging, especially in a society that is crammed with conflicts, tragedies and divergent conclusion. It can be difficult to stay at peace with the people around you, and with the rest of society. Begin by forming bonds with friends and family members, friends, and even your neighbors. Be focused on resolving any conflicts within your life by being kind and compassionate manner and giving an opportunity to those within your community. Also, ensure that you keep your own sense of amiability, which helps you feel at peace with other people.

Method1: Connecting to Others

Participate in events organized by networks. Look through the sheets of your neighborhood network for announcements on events such as the square gathering or carport offer for the network. Participate in network events and donate items or money to community events. This will help you feel more connected to your community. being more connected with your fellow neighbors.

Method 2 Collaborate with your neighbours.

Reach out to people living around your home. Do a thump on their front door and offer them prepared items. Say "hi" at them.. the city. Be kind and tolerant of your neighbors to create a sense of neighborhood.

It is also possible to invite your friends over for dinner or even a drink to get acquainted with them.

Offer to help your neighbors. For instance, if you have a long-time neighbor Offer to help them by helping with their yard or tasks like clearing the gutters.

Step 3.

Spend time with your friends every day. Spend time with good friends so that you are able to remain connected with them and keep in contact. Schedule regular hangouts every week or twice per month with different acquaintances. Make an effort to keep your family ties alive and alive.

For instance, you could organize a coffee break each week with a friend. You could also organize month-to-month game night with a group of friends.

Set up traditions with your loved ones. Consider things like gathering for celebrations of special events or even taking an annual trip with your loved ones.

Step 4

Spend time with your family. Try to make the time you go to with family members is to be important and vital. Enjoy a traditional family dinner or celebrate your family's accomplishments. Make plans for an outing with your loved ones, especially in the event that you've been away for a while because you've all traveled with your family.

If you don't live particularly close to your family You can at least try to get them involved at times. It is possible that the more time you spend with your family members, the more comfortable with your family members you'll grow into.

Take note of your family's traditions and try to create new ones. The sharing of life's events and the recollection of moments shared creates a sense of having a home.

Step 5

You can be a defender and a legit person with family members. Let yourself be open to those you love dearly when you require them. Be sure to not conceal your emotions or keep from sharing your thoughts to them. Instead, remain in the dark so you feel more authentic and real with people around you.

In case you're experiencing a rough day You could say to your friends "Today was a terrible day. I'm in need of some reviving" as well as "I'm not feeling great today. I'm in need of assistance."

Step 6

Be generous and attentive to your partner or friend. Your approach to your relationship is a sentimental one. with respect and affection. Offer them daily consideration and affirmation. Let them know that they are important in your eyes and tell them that you respect them.

It is possible to do this by saying to your companion regularly, "Thank you for all your do" or "I would like to welcome you."

Method 2

Resolving Differences and Disagreements

Avoid shouting or hollering at other people. Take whatever steps you need to avoid to become violent or angry at other people, as it will only exacerbate the conflict. Relax and try to deal with the other person in a measured peaceful manner.

If you're feeling extremely upset If you are extremely disturbed, you could try to escape indefinitely away from the situation and then return later when you're more relaxed and calm.

Recognize the other person's resentment and propose to talk about the situation a bit later. Allow both of you to relax a bit so that you can have a successful conversation that's not overwhelmed by emotions.

2. Respond to anger with compassion and sympathy. Try to respond to any conflict in your life by expressing sympathy and understanding. Instead of expressing anger think about how you can get past

the issue and come up with the solution. Find ways to be a good friend to other people and deal with their shortcomings or concerns instead of trying to change them or help them realize your point of viewpoint.

If, for instance, you find yourself in conflict with someone else, take note of what they might feel about the circumstances. Try to understand the perspective of their partner and then react to them in a way that shows sympathy instead of anger.

Be aware that every event has diverse implications for different people. Make an effort to learn what they are used to through the words, "Assist me with seeing the way you view this particular situation."

3. Be a person who is attentive. Stay in contact with the person with whom you are speaking regardless of whether or not you don't agree with what they're saying. Relax your arms to your sides and move your body toward them so that they can

see your attention is on them. Smile and say "uh-huh" or "OK" to show them that you're listening.

Do not interfere during their conversations. Instead, just wait and wait for them to finish talking. When they are done you can try trying to repeat what they have said to them so that they'll realize that you've were able to hear them.

For example, you could say, "What I think you stated is ..."" "What I've heard you say is ...".

4. Be ready to settle. Sometimes, things don't work out your way. It is possible to find a an agreement with someone that you do not agree with, or release your pride and accept the tradeoff. Accepting a tradeoff could help you move on from the issue and not letting the differences disturb you or cause conflict.

In this instance, for instance, you might find a compromise with your partner in which you share the obligations of the family unit, instead of arguing about these. In contrast you might come to an agreement with a partner in which you work together on a particular task instead of fighting over the length or going in a fight.

Bargain means that both gatherings agree to allow for a portion of what each group requires. Make sure you are prepared to let go some of your possessions with the hope to be positive.

5. Be aware that you won't be in agreement with all. One of the major aspects of living in harmony with other people's perceptions is that you'll not be able to get along with all people you meet. There are many thoughts that limit your thinking or traits that make it difficult to find a common opinion. Be prepared to accept the fact that you may have to come to a compromise with some people within your life.

Even if you don't like an individual or agree with them, isn't a reason to not be able to feel empathy and love for them. It is possible to, in any event, be a part of people you do not agree with and develop a feeling of a sense of comity.

Method 3: Returning to Others

1. Help a friend or a friend to get help for someone who is struggling. Let everyone know that you are concerned by offering the assistance they need when they need it. Don't be a burden for them to seek payment, and you will be comfortable with them.

You might have a friend or relative experiencing sickness or discomfort. Take them to a restaurant when they're too worn out to even think about cooking.

You can assist your neighbor by trying tasks such as scooping snow for them, or taking care of their pets when they go on a trip.

You could also spend time with a partner who is managing the ongoing tension. Encourage them to get better by inviting them to the bar or going on a memorable date night with your companion.

2. Volunteer for a neighborhood association. Find local associations online and other charities in your area that require volunteers. Find a volunteer opportunity to your neighborhood asylum for the destitute or women's safe home. Volunteer your time for an event for charity or the local expressions celebration. By volunteering your time, you can provide you to feel positive connected to others.

Volunteering isalso an amazing way to get to know like-minded people and create new acquaintances or friends. It can help expand your network of group and help you feel less isolated around the globe.

3. Spend money for a noble cause. You could also put your money into a cause

that you trust. Make a donation to a local support group within your area or to a nationwide crusade which focuses on your goals and beliefs.

You can try your hand at donating cash to someone who is a great motivator at least every month, based on your earnings.

4. Become a coach. Find tutoring programs within your local area through the neighborhood network or expressions that focus. Look into your local schools for tutoring programs in which you can are working with children. Try your hand at coaching in a program similar to Big Brother, Big Sister in which you work with a child and move around acting being their teacher.

You could also coach other students as a guide volunteer in an after-school program.

Some graduated class relations in colleges and schools offer mentoring programs for students who want to work professionals in the fields of interest.

5. Check out local businesses. Give back to your local economic development by visiting neighborhood groups within your immediate vicinity. Look for nearby businesses and help them grow by going through your bank account there. Get familiar with local businesses so that you find yourself in cohesion with your local community.

You could, for instance, visit your local market for cattle and become familiar with the vendors who are selling their products there.

Method 4: Maintaining Your Harmony

Keep your sense of Harmony

1. Find a passion or movement that you like. Take time to focus on an interest that you enjoy such as writing, painting, perusing or drawing. It is also possible to play games for fun such as golf, ball or ski.

Maybe you enjoy watching terrible television to calm yourself and relaxing activity.

Engaging in activities you enjoy and do will make you feel more at ease. It will make you feel more relaxed. time, radiate an energy that other are around will be able to sense.

2. Try yoga and deep relaxation. It is possible to experience a state of peace when you are in harmony with your breathing and your body are in sync are in harmony. You can do this by attending classes in your local yoga studio or recreation center. It is also possible to do deep breathing exercises that will assist you in not having a worry about the world.

The profound breathing and yoga practices can also be extremely beneficial to help you focus your mind and feeling more satisfied with yourself and the world around you.

3-.Set aside effort for self-care. Self-care means paying attention to your needs and setting aside time to attend to those needs. You can practice self-care at home, or even trying a few cosmetics. It is also possible to set the time aside to browse or sleep. Engaging in an activity like running or stretching can also be a natural care.

If you're a slave to a busy or unorganized timetable, you should have the idea of putting the time aside for 30 minutes to an hour each day to focus your self-care. Plan it out so that you won't forget it or neglect it.

4. Make use of positive affirmations. Positive affirmations can help in advancing your goals, and those around you , with a sense of peace and generosity. Make positive affirmations in the beginning of the day prior to departing to the afternoon or at night time, before you go to going to bed.

For example, you might say, "I am content with the world" or "I find myself happy and comfortable today."

Be sure to live the way you are by your character. When your approach to life's responsibilities is in line with your personality and thoughts, you'll be less agitated.

Life is an ensemble with low and high points, many awe-inspiring moments as well as triumphal strolls, and instruments that are in an enthralling harmony with each other.

Let me ask you this question: Would you consider yourself content with your amazing outfit? A healthy balance can increase your happiness and success and also your physical health.

Living a happy life is similar to living in a forest with each element having an objective in this huge creature. Every part has a purpose and each of them is connected with each other, dependent on one another's durability.

Here are seven details that will help you continue with a happy life:

1. Live your life with enthusiasm.

The odds of you being born were so low and, yet, you're here. You've been blessed with the most wonderful gift life!

Keep your life a positive example. Be enthusiastic and full of energy. The first thing you do is rise at the beginning of your day and smile at the top of your lungs and say, "It's another extraordinary day to be alive!" Invigorate your motors and massage your body to respect your body and bring harmony and peace for your mind!

Does it really matter if it's not only stunning for you to have a beautiful face? !

2. Show appreciation and gratitude.

As a stream, it encourages the natural environment around it. showing gratitude and appreciation to family and friends. connects you to your family and friends.

Inform them of how important and precious to you they are; how it makes your life better due to having them around.

There are times you might be silent and think about the words you'd like to say, but you don't have the hesitation to say them without fear of fear. The fear that, once the words leave your mouth, maybe your loved ones aren't up to par will not try to portray the amazing people they are.

In fact, it's a real thing it could happen. However, many people don't know regarding your message and investing in more energy.

Thankfulness and appreciation are the blessings that you can give as a result of the vast array of things you receive.

3. Find out how to share.

If you've got an animal, you are aware that conversation is always happening. For instance, your pet does not speak to you, but after you're able to almost make out each other's thoughts. You look at each other.

Many complain that "Our relationship is falling in the wrong direction because we require correspondence. We don't convey." Be aware that you're transmitting something particular every moment when you're in view of someone; perhaps it's not because you're occupied with completing something else.

If your words don't speak through your voice, your body does. Furthermore when you talk the tone of your voice speaks more than the words you speak.

4. Know what you require.

Identify what you need in your daily your life. Be aware of where you're going to ensure you have an organized plan of how to get there. If you don't have even the most basic idea of where to begin you can start by looking at things that are missing from your daily life. What can give meaning and importance to your life?

Be curious about what you are able to accomplish as well as how much more you could do. Be sure to remind yourself that at the end of your life the most important thing to one is the legacy that he or she leaves behind.

5. Have empathy.

Being a good person will require you to do one thing that is to the exclusion of all other things: be compassionate.

Feel empathy for yourself and others. Accept people as they are and tune into the world of discovery that will help you understand and be able to truly see the person in front of you.

Sometimes, the person that you were before will become you. Be aware of the times the moment when things are difficult (for the reasons you) and offer a hug to your inner self. Allow yourself to be excused when you commit mistakes. Accept your impediments as permanent.

Give a final embrace to your soul that is free from guilt, judgement or blame. You and all those around are all just individuals.

6. Teach others how you treat others.

The way you treat yourself determines the precedents for what you expect from other people. Treat yourself with respect. Be pleasant and talk about yourself. You are the guardian of the person you are and the person you must change into. As a lion guards his territory, ensure your self-image, prosperity as well as your the future.

7. Stay positive.

Everything that happens in our lives is positive in some way. Find that positive aspect of life and make sure that no matter what life brings you, you'll find the way to go.

Be aware that there isn't an problem without an answer. Be aware of the possible possibilities open to you.

Take care of your environment the antagonists (individuals or things) and pay attention, observe and see the wonderful aspect of your life.

Chapter 12: Maintaining relationships that use Hygge In Both Your Family and Friends

The most significant things you're going to encounter in Hygge is the concept of family. You won't be able to fully live such a lifestyle without having your family and closest friends to spend time with every day. The people of Denmark believe that people who belong to their families are to be treated with a great deal of respect, concern and affection. For a cozy and comfortable life, ensure that there is some love as much as you can in all the relationships you have with others. We will look at some ways you can add family members, and warmer, to your life.

Make time to reach out to the people you care about

One of the most effective methods you can use to bring this happiness to relationships specifically those that you're trying to build with your family, is you must make the effort to repair relationships that have become strained through the years. If you're not getting along with the people you love living in your life, it's usually due to a dispute or disagreement that occurred with your family or acquaintances. To repair these relationships and assist you in achieving Hygge within your relationship, you may have to take the first step of reaching out to those you cherish.

The first step is to work on making amends with people with whom you've experienced bad relations with over the years. Contact your family member you have problems with, and discuss the issue with them, and bring the fact that you are embarrassed because you were in a disagreement with them or avoided them for a lengthy period of time. In most cases, this will to suffice to assist people feel better and to open the lines of communication , so you can make amends. Making this apology will help allow you to demonstrate to the person that you understand that they have the right to feel at fault for the actions and also lets them look like they're doing something right in their decision to accept your apology. At the end of the day, it could help you both to begin to build an exciting new relationship.

Also, ensure that your loved ones are getting an opportunity to talk about the incident that occurred with you. If any of the relatives decides that they're not willing to accept your apology, know that they've made the decision that they don't wish to have you in their lives at the moment. If you actually took the time to express your apology in a manner that is appropriate and attempted to repair the fence that you had to cross, it could be the only thing you have to do right now. You might have to let it go at this point and be required to continue making amends with your others who are more open.

When you have taken the time to contact those relatives that whom you haven't seen in time, it's an ideal idea to visit them often. If they're some distance away, it's not enough to meet them just every few months. You could decide to take control and create an hyggelig party in your house and hold it a couple of times throughout the year, in addition to the holiday season. It is possible that family members will eventually participate in this and you'll begin being able to connect with relatives more frequently to experience this warm and bonded feeling.

Spending time with people you cherish

In order to experience the warmth and intimacy that is celebrated in relation to Hygge You will have to ensure that you're spending time with your family. You must ensure that you are meeting your family members as well as your acquaintances at least a couple of times a month , if not more. A lot of families during this busy period will only get together just a few times a year with each other, but that does not suffice for them to build the bond you require to be able to enjoy Hygge You must ensure that you spend sufficient time with the people you cherish to assist with the social aspects of your friendships.

How many hours of time spent with loved ones you cherish is sufficient? In the world of Hygge it is suggested that you spend at minimum one hour every day with the person you love. It doesn't have to be difficult. Simple things like eating dinner with your children and your spouse, or reading books in the evening as well as listening to the spouse discuss their day can count in this. Of of course, spending time with your friends and attending larger gatherings could all contribute to this too.

When you're enjoying your time with your loved ones, it is crucial to focus on making good memories. The most enjoyable part of making your own new memories is that you're doing them with people who you truly love and are able to hold them in your heart and the joy you feel whenever you think about this memory, will help you through the difficult time.

If you engage in an activity that is meaningful while you're together with loved ones you'll be creating an unforgettable memory. You can take a trip to the park and enjoy lunch, go fishing, read stories with your children or even watch a hilarious film together. You can be more imaginative should you wish but it could be quite simple to create the memories you desire.

Be peaceful with other people.

If you're with your family and friends it is crucial to make sure that everyone has an agreement at this point. There are occasions when family members and friends may have disagreements with one another however, if you'd prefer a relaxed gathering, it's supposed to be one that isn't a source of many arguments or conflict. If you're gathered in one of these events it is best to seek out a way to bring an end to the conflict and make sure to respect others attending the gathering regardless of what's happening between both of you.

In this gathering, in the event that think there's something that could be causing result in arguments or a disagreement between you and another individual, you'll be required not to bring it up. The discussion of these issues will only cause a negative impact on the gathering without reason. You will find that it's not an easy to ignore these issues at times however, be aware that you're trying to bring happiness to the entire group and this argument is not going to assist any person feel better.

It doesn't have to be a contest

Some gatherings you attend will result in a huge rivalry. Both of you will be spending many hours trying to prove that one person is the superior person, with the most possessions, has the bigger house and more. But this kind of competition isn't likely to make any of you feel more confident. Both sides will be feeling like they are who are being smacked about and neither will be happier, even if they win this battle.

One way you can ensure the members of your family members are having a great time during conversations is to ensure that everyone else can feel at ease in your presence regardless of whether they are in your personal home or at a different one. While the Danes are likely to speak about their fame and goals in certain instances, these will be handled in a way that is not emphasized. They believe that in order to bring Hygge to the table it is necessary to minimize the significance of all these aspects. There's no place for a conversation which will be focused solely on the ambitions or accomplishments of one individual.

Instead, your conversations about hyggelig will help you be a reminder that you've achieved all the goals you'd like to achieve from life, but the best part to consider is it's unlikely that anyone else has achieved this as well. It's not necessary to be talking about things that will make everyone feel down. This doesn't mean you can't gather with your buddies and family to talk about some of your accomplishments or things happening within your own life. However, you'll not be practicing truly Hygge when the other people who are in the discussion share some of similar successes.

One method to ensure that you're making your family members feel at ease around you is to avoid create a sense of competition while you talk. It doesn't matter whether your work is the best in the family or if you own the largest house, and talking about these topics a lot during the discussion is just an attempt to make people feel uncomfortable.

To avoid certain issues in the future, you must be focused on bringing out certain good or exceptional qualities that you recognize in your other family members and acquaintances. Even if you do not consider them in the same way as you do it will help much better when you speak about them. This will make someone else feel better when you discuss the person for a little while and helps bring positive emotions you'd like to see to create in your gatherings. If you're hosting your own hyggelig gatherings refrain from discussing the things you have accomplished and focus on the great things others are doing instead.

Being expressive

We've talked about several of the rules associated with Hygge and the inclusion of them into your family life. But it is also important to spend some time to understand how to communicate the feelings that you feel with the people you appreciate, whether they're one of your friends or family members. If you're not able to express your feelings to them then it's difficult to truly feel comfortable and at ease with them. There are lots of various ways you are capable of doing this type of thing, for example, gifting the family member an extra special present or helping them out and offering a warm word.

People who are in your life are likely to be thrilled when they discover that you offer to lend a hand particularly if you're not seeking any type of reward from this entire process. For starters consider taking a moment to consider ways you can assist the people you love, and especially those who may not expect you to show up and aid them.

That's where your art of being attentive will be a key part of the game. It is essential to stay close enough with your loved ones and family that you can know when they're going need assistance and the best way to assist them. A decision you make for one person isn't always considered an ideal idea for someone else Keep this in mind while you're observing and trying to determine what each person needs from you.

Additionally, you must spend some time to think about the ways you can act to let the people you love how much you love them. In the present there is a tendency that you will overlook the people you love to the core. However, this could make them feel uneasy and could result in some conflicts between you. You should take some time each day to let your partner know how important they are in your life and truly value them within your lives.

There's a good thing that there are quite many ways you can express your love to those whom you love. It is possible to use the phone, call and assist those who need help in any way, send an email, sending them a present (especially one that is handmade) or come up with a method that has an emotional connection to the person you are in contact with will demonstrate your love them in a unique way.

When it comes to pursuing Hygge and incorporating it into your lifestyle, there is nothing more essential than the concept of family and people whom you cherish. It is crucial to repair any fractured fences that have been erected over time , and you must to be able to spend time with them every day. You'll find that it is not uncommon for people to feel lonely and not be concerned about other people However, humans are social creatures, and if we are to fully enjoy Hygge it is essential to understand that friends and family must be a vital element of our lives. If you're looking to embrace some of the wonderful friendships that are built with your family and friends and are ready to see the results from Hygge Utilize the advice in this chapter to assist you!

Chapter 13: Ten winter tips

As the winter months approach you will naturally be a bit depressed at the thought of colder temperatures and the lack of brightness and color. If this is the case for your situation, then you'll want to be aware of what it takes to Hygge.

In the very first chapter of this small Hygge guide, it was noticed that certain countries like Sweden, Norway, and Denmark during winter only get a few hours of sunlight each day. These are the societies which have developed strategies to live in the time of darkness and darkness. Even if you don't reside in the north, at times the changes in the seasons can be detrimental to your life.

Let's review 10 tips to help you stay warm during the winter months. Like the American Thanksgiving it is a time to be Hygge. Keep in mind these tips you can incorporate into your imagination and family traditions.

The art of writing can provide therapeutic benefits in any way. In the winter months you can sit down with some paper and pen authentic letters to family or friends that live in various places. What would they think of to receive a personal letter from you? Writing a journal and creating poetry are enjoyable ways to relax during the winter months. One book I'd recommend for this moment would be The Artist Way by Julia Cameron.

Turn your home into a day spa. Invite your friends to join you to enjoy a relaxing night of facial treatments. If the products you use are homemade it is Hygge certainly. Winter can dry hair and skin very quickly, and wearing a hat does not help either.

They are always cozy and enjoyable. Bonfires are a great way to create unforgettable and memorable memories especially following The Christmas Holiday.

Invite your friends to bring their dry-out Christmas Trees, wreaths and garland, and then light them up. If you're still enjoying the festive spirit you can include marshmallows and hot dogs to roast. The sharing of holiday stories is always enjoyable and educational. Isn't everyone a family member who acts irrational at Christmas?

Music is Hygge at any season, and it's always fun to sing the songs from your childhood. Bring your family together and allow everyone to talk about their favorite songs. Children, if they are allowed could share music that you're not expecting however they'll be grateful for you taking time to listen.

Set up a weekly task you like, whether it's a time that you cook, sew or creating craft projects. Making Christmas presents with your friends is a great way to have fun and Hygge. The process of putting together an entire church or neighborhood cookbook is extremely enjoyable and can be used as a fundraising tool for local charities.

Plan your week's schedule by and eliminate anything that is technological. Switch off your television or cell phones as well as computers when you eat dinner and converse. If you are a fan of table games this could be the ideal setting to spend time with family members and telling them you appreciate spending time with them.

The movie night could be Hygge if you select the best one. You can create a theater experience for your guests and family by providing boxes of popcorn, film snacks and soft drinks. Print movie tickets that include the time the show will start and the film that is scheduled to be played and place them that they can locate them easily. You should have pillows and blankets on hand to allow your guests to enjoy a relaxing Hygge night.

Plan an Christmas Tree Decorating Party for your family members and perhaps one or two close friends however, keep it private. Serve hot chocolate and other snacks. It is a bit of preparation but you'll require all ornaments as well as the lights and garland to be set to go on the tree. Searching for hooks or working with lighting that is tangled can take the Hygge completely out of the space. You can play Christmas music and soften the mood by using candles with scents, particularly one with a cinnamon or pine fragrance. Make sure everyone wears their favorite Christmas hat, however it is possible to have a few more available for those who feel it's not essential.

Get the kids together and take them to the car to go on a tour of the city's Christmas lights. Numerous cities, neighborhoods and churches get their lights up to celebrate Christmas. It is definitely a Hygge-like experience. It could also be a great night to eat pizza after you return home , or an opportunity to dine in a restaurant you love. Add reindeer antlers on the front of the windows of your vehicle, or the red Rudolf nose on the hood's front can make the celebration more memorable. They are available at nearly every department store in town cheaply.

Plan a night of mulled wines and a swap of sweaters. Chances are that if you're contemplating an Hygge lifestyle, you're someone who has some knitted clothes in the closet. Invite your friends to your home and have them bring their old knits or buy a few from a thrift store. The process of trying on these clothes can be enjoyable and very enjoyable. If you decide to host this in December, it might be themed around Christmas too. There are people who are doing the same thing using the hats. An Hygge Home Hat Party could be a great opportunity to make your friends more interested in the Hygge way of living.

These winter-related tips can be entertaining, but they're also activities that bring families and friends closer in the most difficult season of all. Take advantage of Hygge and transform your home into a sanctuary of winter peace and wellbeing are the most important factor to happiness. Our lives are full of moments that are special which is why you should make every single one of them worth the effort. Hygge is a method to make even the most bleak of days. Hopefully these tips will in establishing living a more comfortable and relaxed life.

Conclusion

Next, begin seeking out ways you can incorporate Hygge into your everyday life. It is a great method to feel content in your life and gain some of the positive items you're searching for to be satisfied and at peace with the world. Many times, we worry about what other people think of us. We're always in a hurry and trying to acquire more things and this isn't the best way to feel happy and be content with the present.

The guidebook takes time to study the concept of Hygge and what it could be to you. It is a wonderful concept to follow since it can help you discover how to be satisfied with what you are able to enjoy and also to surround yourself with people who can bring satisfaction and lots of pleasure. If you're looking to reap the great benefits associated from Hygge be sure to go through this book and discover ways to incorporate the concept to your life.

www.ingramcontent.com/pod-product-compliance
Lightning Source LLC
Chambersburg PA
CBHW060329030426
42336CB00011B/1263